A PICTURE OF HEALTH

THE KEY TO RECEIVING HEALING

kate forsyth

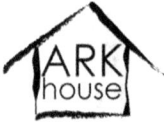

Ark House Press
PO Box 1722, Port Orchard, WA 98366 USA
PO Box 1321, Mona Vale NSW 1660 Australia
PO Box 318 334, West Harbour, Auckland 0661 New Zealand
arkhousepress.com

Cataloguing in Publication Data:
Author: Forsyth, Kate
Title: A Picture of Health
ISBN: 9780987388834 (pbk.)
Subjects: Spiritual healing | Spiritual biography
Dewey Number: 234.131

Cover design and layout by initiateagency.com

ENDORSEMENTS

If you have ever needed healing in your own life , or in someone close to you-or desire to see healings through your own prayers-you will LOVE this book by Pastor Kate. Like the author, Kate-I have witnessed personal healing and seen it in others. There is nothing more amazing than being privy to Gods healing touch.

All healing is miraculous! Whether through medical intervention, healthy lifestyle changes, and the divine intervention through prayer.

Some believers have been given the gift of healing. Kate is one such minister. She has witnessed miracles in her own life-and this has developed, along with her husband Richard-into a deep desire to release it to others.

I believe there is a new kind of minister who releases Gods healing power. Not on a vast stage with music, bells and whistles-but quietly through the homes, schools, streets and businesses of everyday life. In kitchens, cafes, shops and in small gatherings of believers. The prayer of faith is saving the sick. I see an army of supernatural practitioners-not weird or flashy-but anointed everyday believers "going about doing good-and healing all who are oppressed by the devil".

Kate is one such believer.

I know as you read this book-faith will rise in your heart-you will begin to witness Gods healing grace and power, not only in your life-but others too.

Chris Pringle
Senior Minister C3 Church

Kate Forsyth has been a part of the C3 College teaching faculty for 15 years, and over this time has powerfully impacted many lives with her clear and relevant Bible teaching. The stand out over this time has been Kate's teaching on healing. Coming from a background of personal experience and revelation in the area of healing, and with an understanding of what the Bible says about healing, has allowed Kate to see the most extraordinary results in this area in her students lives. Not only have students received healing for themselves, they have been equipped to minister healing to others. I am confident that this book will bring the same outcome for you, and the people around you.

Pat Antcliff
Principal, C3 College

CONTENTS

ACKNOWLEDGEMENTS

I want to thank my beautiful family, Richard my wonderful husband and my two amazing miracles, our children, Annalise and Michael. Thank you for all your encouragement over the years, your belief in me and for being the incredible people that you are.

I want to also thank our pastors, Phil and Chris Pringle, who have always been such an inspiration to myself and my family. You are so full of faith, full of love for God and always leading us onwards in all that He has for us. Thank you for the foundation of faith that you placed in our lives over the years and your incredible example of godly, faith filled lives - we wouldn't be the people that we are without your amazing leadership, faith, vision and encouragement.

Thank you to Helen Reardon for sharing her testimony in how she received healing through Communion.

Thank you to Jane Allen, who in obeying the Lord in a seemingly small thing, helped so much in changing a big thing in our lives.

Thank you also to Brett Barclay, Helen Reardon, Naomi Henshall, Helen Manning and Katie Haldane for proof reading the book for me.

Thank you to all the people who have encouraged me to write down the healing course that I have taught for years. There are too many to list (so my apologies for not doing so) but special mention to Wendy Gilbert, Helen Manning, Merry Watson and Heidi Wysman.

Thank you to the myriad of teachers of faith who, over the years, have each contributed a little piece of understanding, a piece to the puzzle, that has grown into in a wonderful picture of what Jesus has done for us.

Above all else, thank you to Jesus, our God and Saviour, who made miraculous healing a reality and gift to us all, through an unimaginable price that He paid on our behalf.

INTRODUCTION

This book comes out of a passion to see the eyes of believers opened to the extraordinary salvation that Jesus has provided for us and, in doing so, that healing has been provided for us as much as the forgiveness of sins. It is written with the aim to help people appropriate God's healing for themselves and also be able to minister it.

Healing seems to be one of the greatest areas of unbelief, contention and resistance in the church today, and yet, is an area so important to God, that He went to extraordinary lengths to provide it for us.

This book by no means covers every aspect of the Lord's healing grace nor every scripture relating to it, but rather, what He has enlightened to me in my own journey towards healing. My prayer is that it will help you also, if you are on that journey or you would like to help others who are.

All Bible scriptures will be in "The New King James" version, unless specified otherwise.

HOW IT ALL BEGAN

Even before I came to know Jesus, I had a hunger to understand how to heal the sick. This had previously lead me on a journey studying pharmacy and then, looking into all the natural therapies. While I hold the medical world in the highest esteem, there are also areas of frustration that arise where some ailments are difficult to heal, some impossible, and some at huge expense to the patient.

Prior to becoming a Christian, I had experienced a lifetime of illness from a poor immune system. This poor health was aggravated when I became anorexic in my late teens. In the three years preceding meeting Christ, I sustained a severe back injury from a car accident and a horse riding accident that left me with excruciating pain, severe headaches daily and being unable to move my neck from side to side. My husband, then boyfriend, Richard also had a severe back injury from an accident in the mining industry and so, twice each week, we would both be visiting chiropractors and physiotherapists (very romantic!). Over the years, the pain was not getting better, but worse.

On the 26th February, 1989, I walked into Christian City Church at Brookvale, Sydney (now C3 Church, Oxford Falls) and felt an amazing sense of life, not knowing at the time that, this life was God Himself. I decided to check out the service that day and come back later, to make a decision about becoming a Christian. During the week that followed, I had such a sense of excitement and anticipation about the following Sunday and couldn't wait for it to come around. On the 5th March, I asked Jesus Christ to come into my life. What I didn't realise at the time was that I was not just receiving forgiveness of sins that day but

I was asking The Healer to come into my life, my body, and that He was intent on removing my sickness as well as my sins.

At first, I wasn't aware of just how much Jesus had done, until in the days and weeks ahead I realised that all pain had left my body, the headaches had stopped and I could now move my neck from side to side. The power of anorexia was completely broken and I felt a strong inner voice that I was to eat well and not worry, not calorie count or restrict my food intake in the way that I had been doing for years. I was also delivered from an overwhelming sense of fear and anxiety that I had lived with all my life.

Two weeks after my decision, Richard also asked Christ into his life and went from having to rely on having access to a chiropractor wherever he went, to complete healing of his back and removal of all pain. In the months ahead for me it became apparent that the healing had gone way beyond the back injury, to the rest of my body. Having previously had a deficient immune system, I would go through winters with constant colds, a few doses of the 'flu and then sinus and hay fever problems the rest of the year, along with other immune problems. I had also regularly suffered cold sores, but not as most people do with a single sore on the mouth. Since the age of six I had experienced them in my eyes, called herpes keratitis, which had significantly affected my eyesight. I would also get extensive outbreaks over my face, covering my skin, the nose area and all around the mouth, whenever I had been stressed, which was often. Suddenly, I was well and all of these conditions had left my body.

One of the leaders of the connect group that we attended, introduced me to the truth about God's healing power. I was so excited to have found the way that the sick would be healed. The following six months were amazing as we saw God move in every area of our lives, bringing His blessing and turning around circumstances that had been against us. During that time, whenever a headache or pain would come, a quick prayer was all that was needed and it would miraculously go. I was naively thinking to myself, "This healing is so easy!"

However, a week after we were married in December that year, I started to feel really unwell. I continued to pray and 'just get on with it' but, by May the following year, I had a physical breakdown following an autoimmune disease that I had basically just let go too far without addressing the increasing symptoms. As a result, every organ in my body was shutting down. My heart dangerously slowed, my digestive system packed it in, I was jaundiced as my liver function dropped and I was so physically weak that I could only move around for about ten minutes before needing an hour's rest. My brain function was so poor that I couldn't interpret what people were saying to me, nor put words together to respond. People would ask how I was and I couldn't even put those simple words together and would have to say, "I'm sorry. I don't understand".

In addition, we received a medical report that told us that we would be unlikely to be able to have children due to a severe case of polycystic ovaries with which I had no ovulation, the damage from the years of anorexia and the autoimmune disease that caused miscarriages. We were advised that we should be looking at fertility support or IVF. Being a scientist and having a love of seeing how things work, and the need to see things work rather than just going on the words of others, I decided that this was a prime opportunity to see God do the impossible.

This lead me on a discovery in the Word of God about the healing that God has provided for us and how we receive it, so that it's not just a lovely theory but a living reality.

Like any baby, a new Christian finds everything comes easily to them, but like any parent, God wants us to grow up from there and learn how to relate to Him and receive from Him through faith.

I find that there is a lot of confusion in believers about the teaching surrounding faith and how to actually live it out. It is my hope that in the following pages to simplify that process. I make no apology for the amount of scripture that will be covered, as the life of God is not only found in His Spirit but in His Word and this life is healing to us. I have found that in every situation we faced, God highlighted different scriptures to us and so in including many of them, I believe that there will be some that the reader will find speaks to them.

So as you read on, I pray 'that the God of our Lord Jesus Christ, the Father of glory, may give to you the spirit of wisdom and revelation in the knowledge of Him, the eyes of your understanding being enlightened; that you may know what is the hope of His calling, what are the riches of the glory of His inheritance in the saints, and <u>what is the exceeding greatness of His power toward us who believe…</u>' (Ephesians 1:17-19).

1

ESTABLISHING A SCRIPTURAL FOUNDATION FOR HEALING

....

Before starting on how to receive healing, I want to spend a couple of chapters to lay a foundation for biblical healing and to create a basis for faith. Without faith it is not only impossible to please God (Hebrews 11:6) but it is unlikely to receive His promises. The promises of God are given by grace and received through faith and Romans 10:17 tells that *'faith comes by hearing and hearing by the word of God'*. So, we need to know what the Word of God says on a matter in order to be in a place of faith.

For faith to operate, you must know Who you believe, what you believe and why you believe it. It must be so established in your heart that it can stand under opposition, persecution and challenges to its validity. It is not enough to merely believe because someone tells you to. For this reason, I have included much scripture in this book and I encourage you to study the verses and see their truth for yourself.

God's will for mankind has remained the same since the Garden of Eden, where Adam had all his needs met, there was no sickness, he had unbroken fellowship with God and had dominion in the Earth. God's will was done on earth as it is in heaven. There was no sickness in the Garden of Eden prior to the fall of man.

In the chapter on 'Healing in Redemption', we will see that sin allowed sickness to come into the human race and has been present ever since. This does not mean that if someone is sick, that it is because of some sin in their life but that the origin of sickness in mankind came through sin. What we will find is that Jesus dealt with sickness at the same time that He dealt with our sins.

From the time of man's fall God has had to provide healing for His people because all of mankind has had to deal with this issue. We see throughout scripture that God has always provided healing for those who come to Him in faith because it is His will for us to be well.

3 John 2

Beloved I pray that you may prosper in all things and be in health, just as your soul prospers.

God revealed His will to heal His people way back in Exodus, when He established a covenant with the Old Testament believers, to keep them well.

Exodus 15:26

...and said, "If you diligently heed the voice of the LORD your God and do what is right in His sight, give ear to His commandments and keep all His statutes, I will put none of the diseases on you which I have brought on the Egyptians. For I am the LORD who heals you."

The translation of 'the Lord who heals you' is 'Jehovah Rapha'. The names of the Lord starting with Jehovah, in the Old Testament, are called His redemptive names. Through them, God reveals to His people what He was going to restore to them, that had originally been lost in the fall, in this case health.

The word 'rapha', according to Strong's concordance, means 'to cure, heal, repair, mend, restore health'[2]. It is used in the Bible for the healing of physical sickness, not spiritual.

This scripture models a pattern for receiving healing. God's people are called to position themselves to hear and take heed to His Word and then to do it. Romans 10:17 tells us that *'so then faith comes by hearing, and hearing by the word of God'*. When we attentively listen to the word, faith comes, and then as we act on that faith, we position ourselves to be in a place where God's healing is released to us.

Exodus 23:25, 26

"So you shall serve the LORD your God, and He will bless your bread and your water. And I will take sickness away from the midst of you. No one shall suffer miscarriage or be barren in your land; I will fulfil the number of your days."

God's will for our life is to serve Him, be blessed, free from sickness and the number of our days fulfilled. Psalm 91:16 says, *'with long life will I satisfy you and show you my salvation'*. It is not God's will for you to die early. It is His will for sickness to be removed from you.

Deuteronomy 7:15

"And the LORD will take away from you all sickness, and will afflict you with none of the terrible diseases of Egypt which you have known, but will lay them on all those who hate you."

In Psalm 103, King David reveals the benefits of salvation under the old covenant, as he understood it.

Psalm 103:1-5

Bless the Lord, O my soul;
And all that is within me, bless His holy name!
Bless the Lord, O my soul,
And forget not all His benefits;
Who forgives all your iniquities,
Who heals all your diseases;
Who redeems your life from destruction,
Who crowns you with loving kindness and tender mercies;
Who satisfies your mouth with good things;
So that your youth is renewed like the eagle's.

This is our salvation! We have forgiveness of all sins, healing from all sicknesses, redemption from destruction and the gift of eternal life, God's kindness and mercy, provision and restoration of life.

Verse 5 of Psalm 103 in the Amplified version reads '*Who satisfies your mouth (your necessity and desire at your personal age and situation) with good so that your youth, renewed, is like the eagle's (strong, overcoming, soaring)'*.[3]

So often you hear Christians say that God will only provide your needs but here it says that He provides your desires as well, and then says according to your personal age and situation. This is because your desires and needs are different at different ages and situations in life.

This passage was highlighted to me when my son, Michael was four years of age. This testimony doesn't relate to healing but showed me just how much God wants to meet our desires as well as needs.

When Michael was four, he was crazy about the movie Toy Story, and especially the characters of Woody and Buzz Lightyear. We had bought him toys of both the characters but the one that he really had his heart set on was a large toy of Buzz Lightyear that said a lot of his phrases from the movie. I had considered the larger toy out of our budget and had bought a mid-size one but it was obvious that he still wanted the large one.

One day, I was at my desk studying the Bible and I felt the Holy Spirit clearly say to me to go to Toys R Us, a large toy store at a local shopping centre. I was under the impression that the Lord had someone for me to speak to, some divine encounter. When I reached the store, I felt led to the aisle with the Toy Story toys and my eyes were directed to the Buzz Lightyear toys.

There were three of the special Buzz toys left and two I saw were tampered with and looked like they might be broken. At that moment, a store attendant walked past and said, "those are the last ones anywhere". This was an unusual action, I thought, for someone just walking past a browsing customer. I picked up the last intact toy of this particular Buzz, but immediately my reasoning kicked in.

The reasoning went like this, "he is four years old; he doesn't need one this big and certainly not this expensive; this is not being wise with our budget; he has a Buzz toy, he should be content with that". As I stood reasoning, I felt the Lord speak to me again, "This is the one that he wants; he is My son and I want him to have it".

How often do we consider that God would only be interested in the so-called important things and not be concerned with the desires of our hearts or even just the trivial aspects of our lives. I learnt that day that the God of the universe is concerned that a little boy had the toy that was the desire of his heart, a desire that would only last for a few years and have absolutely no lasting or eternal significance. If God is so concerned about such a small thing, how could He be accused of not being concerned about the important things that we face in life?

God provides for both our needs and desires at our given age and situation, both of which will change. The desire of a little boy is very different to the desire of a young person looking at his or her first car, or the desire of newlyweds looking at their first house or someone else planning a longed for holiday. For others, there will be more important desires such as being able to provide for a family or to be healed from a serious illness. Whatever the need or desire, God is waiting to provide for it if we will trust Him with it. He can be trusted with our desires; He is good in every way and will only bring us good.

James 1:17
Every good and perfect gift is from above, coming down from the Father of lights, with whom there is no variation or shadow of turning.

So we can see that healing was provided under the old covenant but Hebrews 7:22 tells us that *'Jesus has become a surety of a better covenant'*. If healing was provided under the old, then surely it must be part of the new and better covenant.

In the New Testament (or covenant), God's will is revealed through Jesus. Hebrews 1:3 says that Jesus is *'the express image of His person'* (the Father's). In John 7:16 Jesus said *"My doctrine is not Mine but His Who sent Me"*. In response to Phillip asking Jesus to show them the Father, Jesus said in John 14:9, *"he who has seen Me has seen the Father"*.

Hebrews 1:1-3

God, who at various times and in various ways spoke in time past to the fathers by the prophets, has in these last days spoken to us by His Son, whom He has appointed heir of all things, through whom also He made the worlds; who being the brightness of His glory <u>and the express image of His person,</u> and upholding all things by the word of His power, when He had by Himself purged our sins, sat down at the right hand of the Majesty on high,

In John 14:10 and John 5:17-21, Jesus tells us that the Father who dwelt in Him did His works; the words He spoke were His Father's words and what He did was the result of what He saw His Father do. Thus, Jesus is the revelation of God in all He says and does.

Now the book of John goes on to reveal that Jesus was not just the image of the Father but was God Himself in the flesh.

John 1:1-4

In the beginning was the Word, and <u>the Word was with God, and the Word was God</u>. He was in the beginning with God. All things were made through Him, and without Him nothing was made that was made. In Him was life, and the life was the light of men.

John 1:14

And the Word became flesh and dwelt among us, and we beheld His glory, the glory as of the only begotten of the Father, full of grace and truth.

Therefore, we see Jesus the Word, with God the Father and the Holy Spirit in the beginning. The Bible teaches that God is the union of three divine Persons in one Godhead, called the Trinity-the Father, the Son or the Word (as Jesus was known before coming to earth), and the Holy Spirit; and these three are co-equal and co-eternal.

Genesis 1:26a

Then God said "Let <u>Us</u> make man in <u>Our</u> image, according to Our likeness."

Isaiah 6:8

Also I heard the voice of the Lord saying "Whom shall I send, and who will go for <u>Us</u>?"

1 John 5:7

For there are three that bear witness in heaven: the Father, the Word, and the Holy Spirit; and <u>these three are one</u>.

Referring to the passages in John (1:1-4, 14), all things were made through the Word (John 1:12, Colossians 1:16,17). The Word, the second Person of the Trinity, came into Mary's womb and became flesh, being born into this earth as Jesus. God is Spirit and so when the Word of God came into Mary's womb, He came as a spirit. Jesus' spirit was the Word of God (the second Person of the Trinity) and He had a human body and soul (without the sin nature). This is how He was both man and God. He was manifested as a man so that He could identify with humanity and be a spotless sacrifice before God the Father, in order to remove man's sin. After His resurrection, He then returned to Heaven to dwell with the Father as the Word of God again. In Revelation 19:13, describing the Second Coming of Christ, we see that He is called the Word of God.

In **John 17:5**, Jesus says, *"And now, O Father, glorify Me together with Yourself, with the glory which I had with You before the world was."*

John reveals that Jesus is God Himself. Therefore, if we want to know what the will of God is, we just have to look at Jesus' ministry and what His priorities were. The gospels reveal that a large part of Jesus' ministry was healing the sick. Did this healing pass away when Jesus returned to Heaven?

Hebrews 13:8

Jesus Christ is the same yesterday, today, and forever.

This means that God is the same yesterday, today and forever. God does not change His character or nature with time. In **Malachi 3:6** God says, *"I am the Lord, I do not change"*. He is still the Healer.

Looking at a couple of examples of Jesus' response to people seeking healing, we see that He is not just able to heal us but is willing to heal us.

Matthew 8:2, 3

And behold, a leper came and worshiped Him, saying, "Lord, if You are willing, You can make me clean."

Then Jesus put out His hand and touched him, saying, "I am willing; be cleansed." Immediately his leprosy was cleansed.

Matthew 8:5-7

Now when Jesus had entered Capernaum, a centurion came to Him, pleading with Him, saying, "Lord, my servant is lying at home paralyzed, dreadfully tormented."

And Jesus said to him, "I will come and heal him."

The following are some passages relating to Jesus ministry which obviously reveal God's will for us. If God came to earth, what would be His priority in His message to mankind? God did come to earth and His message was to show people how to have a relationship with Himself and others, and to demonstrate His will in healing the sick, casting out demons and raising the dead.

Matthew 9:35, 36

Then Jesus went about all the cities and villages, teaching in their synagogues, preaching the gospel of the kingdom, and healing every sickness and every disease among the people. But when He saw the multitudes, He was moved with compassion for them, because they were weary and scattered, like sheep having no shepherd.

Matthew 8:16, 17

When evening had come, they brought to Him many who were demon-possessed. And He cast out the spirits with a word, and

healed all who were sick, that it might be fulfilled which was spoken by Isaiah the prophet, saying:
"He Himself took our infirmities
And bore our sicknesses."

Mark 6:56

Wherever He entered, into villages, cities, or the country, they laid the sick in the marketplaces, and begged Him that they might just touch the hem of His garment. And as many as touched Him were made well.

Matthew 15:30, 31

Then great multitudes came to Him, having with them the lame, blind, mute, maimed, and many others; and they laid them down at Jesus' feet, and He healed them. So the multitude marvelled when they saw the mute speaking, the maimed made whole, the lame walking, and the blind seeing; and they glorified the God of Israel.

Luke 4:40

When the sun was setting, all those who had any that were sick with various diseases brought them to Him; and He laid His hands on every one of them and healed them.

Luke 6:17-19

And He came down with them and stood on a level place with a crowd of His disciples and a great multitude of people from all Judea and Jerusalem, and from the seacoast of Tyre and Sidon, who came to hear Him and be healed of their diseases, as well as those who were tormented with unclean spirits. And they were healed. And the whole multitude sought to touch Him, for power went out from Him and healed them all.

Healing was the 'calling card' of Jesus' ministry. Later, in discussing faith, we will see that hearing the Word is important in receiving healing. With reaching those who do not yet know the Lord, healing is important in them hearing and receiving the Word. Healings may not bring faith but they do bring hope. When people see God's mercy in healing, it gives them hope for His forgiveness, which they can't see. Many people won't hear the gospel but if they have an encounter with God and are healed, then they will hear. In Jesus' ministry, it is recorded that *'they came to hear and be healed'* (Luke 6:17).

It is the goodness of God that leads man to repentance (Romans 2:4). Often people have to see His goodness before they will repent. The following are two examples of my experience with this.

The first was with a person who we had been praying for and were asking to our fellowship group, in our church called a 'connect group'. We tried for a long time to no avail. Finally one night she came after the message, indicating that she would just have a cup of tea so that she could say that she had come. She happened to have a broken foot which lead the conversation to healing and I asked if I could pray for her foot. Another member of the group and myself prayed, and the lady's foot was healed. After that, she attended our group regularly. She came to hear because she had been healed.

Another incident that stands out is when my husband Richard prayed for a lady. This particular lady didn't like church, thought we were all crazy (in her words) and would never have come, but she had called the church to help a friend of hers who was in trouble. In the course of a conversation, it came out that she had suffered from a bleeding issue for about two months with fibrotic cysts. Richard said he would pray for her.

Telling me the story the following week, she said that she was driving at the time and had her hand that was holding the phone out of the window so that she couldn't hear the prayer, saying, "Who is this nutter?" When she got home she realised that she had been healed. The following week I was talking with her at church, and she was alternating between, 'I don't know what I am doing here; I think Christians are nutters; this is all weird', to 'all I know is, I got healed'.

That lady was to go on to become a believer and be established in church. She didn't come because someone preached at her; she came because she was healed and experienced the goodness of

God. Healing opens people's hearts to hear the gospel that will bring their ultimate healing.

The apostle Paul says of his ministry in 1 Corinthians 2:4, 5, *'And my speech and my preaching <u>were not with persuasive words of human wisdom</u> but in <u>demonstration of the Spirit and power</u>, that your faith should not be in the wisdom of men, but in the power of God.'*

PICTURE

SEE IT FOR YOUR LIFE!

GOD IS YOUR HEALER

HE REMOVES ALL SICKNESS FROM YOU

HE HEALS ALL YOUR DISEASES

HE IS WILLING TO HEAL YOU

2

HOW SICKNESS CAME TO MANKIND

....

To understand the remedy for sickness, we first need to look at how it entered the world, because God always deals with the root cause of a thing and not just the symptoms.

Romans 5:12
Therefore, just as through one man sin entered the world, and death through sin, and thus death spread to all men, because all sinned...

In Genesis 3, when Adam sinned by disobeying God, sin entered the world and death with it. Prior to Adam's sin, there was no sickness, no curse and no death.

In Genesis 2:15-17, God only gave Adam one commandment, to not eat of the tree of the knowledge of good and evil. Some people ask why God would put something in man's world that he couldn't have and that, when wrongly chosen, would bring such devastating results. If everything was perfect and done for us, we would just be like robots, and not children of God with choices. God wanted a people who would choose Him and not just have Him and His blessings by default. For this reason, God will always allow alternative choices in our lives so that we have to choose His way over the way of self or sin. Choosing His way brings great reward.

Genesis 2:15-17
Then the Lord God took the man and put him in the garden of Eden to tend and keep it. And the Lord God commanded the man,

saying, "Of every tree of the garden, you may freely eat; but of the tree of the knowledge of good and evil you shall not eat, for in the day that you eat of it you shall surely die."

The word knowledge here, I have heard taught as meaning 'to know by observing or reflecting (to see or think about) or to know by experience'. God did not want man to experience evil. Note that Eve was not yet created when the command was given.

In Genesis 3:1-6 Satan comes in the form of a serpent, using his main strategies, to create doubt in the Word of God and bring deception. If he can make you doubt or deceive you then he can lead you to sin, and sin is his entry point into the human life.

Genesis 3:1

Now the serpent was more cunning than any beast of the field which the Lord God had made. And he said to the woman, Has God indeed said, 'You shall not eat of every tree of the garden'?"

Satan can't stop you being healed or blessed; he can only tempt you to doubt or sin so that you will not be in a position of faith to receive from God.

All the promises of God are given by grace, and received through faith (Ephesians 2:8; 2 Corinthians 1:20). In Romans 4:16, Paul writes, *'therefore it is of faith that it might be according to grace, so that the promise might be sure to all the seed.'* God has established things so that all of His promises are given by His grace, and not according to our efforts. So all the glory belongs to Him and there is no place for us to get into a place of pride, thinking that we have brought about His goodness by our efforts. He then established that His promises would be received through faith, thus ensuring that these promises would then be guaranteed to all.

```
                God's blessings
                on the path      →  Pressure from the devil
                -given by grace     - doubt, deception and
                                    discouragement to get
                                    you out of faith & off the
                                    path and
                                 →  temptation to get you
                                    into disobedience & off
                                    the path

Position yourself
on the path by                      Promises
Faith and                           received through
Obedience      ──────→|←──────      Faith
```

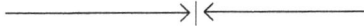

God's path is His will for your life. It is His overriding will for all believers, which includes all the promises that Jesus secured for us by His death and resurrection, and His individual plan for each of our lives. We position ourselves on God's path by our faith in Him and His Word, and by being obedient to His Word and the leading of the Holy Spirit.

God's promises, including healing, are accessed on that path of His will. Our problem is not trying to get God's promises (because they are given freely by grace), but to position ourselves on His path where we can <u>receive</u> them.

Getting onto that path is contested by spiritual forces and sometimes by well-meaning people. The devil will try to knock you off that path by the temptation to sin and by bringing doubt, in God's faithfulness and His Word, deception, and discouragement when it's taking longer than you thought it would. These are designed by the enemy to get you out of a position where you can receive God's blessing. If you understand this, then you can be more aggressive in dealing with doubt and temptation when they come.

Note that in Genesis 3 Satan goes to Eve first, the one who received the Word of God second-hand, because the command given in Genesis 2:16,17 was given to Adam before Eve was created. It is so important that we have revelation of the Word of God for ourselves. We can't receive from God on someone else's revelation and the one who only has the Word second- hand is open to deception.

1Timothy 2:13, 14

For Adam was formed first, then Eve. And Adam was not deceived, but the woman being deceived, fell into transgression.

Firstly Satan comes with doubt, 'Has God indeed said'? Then he moves onto deception, contradicting what God had said with "you will not surely die". Now Eve was deceived, but Adam who was standing by her side throughout the whole scenario, made a deliberate act of disobeying God and hence, sin is said to come through Adam.

Genesis 3:4,5

Then the serpent said to the woman, "You will not surely die. For God knows that in the day you eat of it your eyes will be opened, and you will be like God, knowing good and evil."

Satan tempts by making sin look attractive and that you would be missing out if you did not follow the temptation. You have to remember that the only thing that God was trying to withhold from mankind, with His commandment, was evil. Up to this point, Adam and Eve had only known good. When we look at the Bible, it is not to be seen as a set of restrictive rules and regulations to give you a limited life. It is a structure of how to live in relationship with God and have the incredible and blessed life that He originally intended for you. For this to happen, He calls us to live within boundaries that keep us on His blessed path and away from evil.

Now Genesis 2:17 told us that *'in the day that you eat of it you shall surely die'*, but Genesis 5:5, that Adam lived 930 years. He did not die physically at the moment that they ate from the tree, but he did die spiritually, which is to be separated from God. When God made Adam, He made his body out of the dust of the earth and then breathed His very Spirit into Adam to give him life. It is the spirit of man that is created in the image of God and where the life of God dwells. God is Spirit (John 4:24) and Adam's contact with God was spirit to Spirit. When Adam sinned, God removed Himself and that contact was broken. God is holy and cannot be connected with sin. This separation from God is spiritual death which leads to eventual physical death, with sickness being part of that process.

Genesis 5:1-3

This is the book of the genealogy of Adam. In the day that God created man, He made him in the likeness of God. He created them male and female, and blessed them and called them Mankind in the day they were created. And Adam lived one hundred and thirty years, and begot a son in his own likeness, after his image, and named him Seth.

To clarify a common challenge to this scripture, Adam lived 130 years before he had his son, but his lifespan was 930 years, as recorded in verse five. Adam's son was created, not in the image of God, but in the image of Adam who now had a sin nature and was not in the same unlimited connection with God, and thus the sin nature was perpetuated to all mankind. This is why **Romans 5:12** says *'Therefore, just as through one man sin entered the world, and death through sin, and so death spread to all men because all sinned.'*

Adam's sin brought a new law into the earth. A scientific law is one that produces reproducible results every time that it is put into practice, under the same conditions, such as the law of gravity. The process of sin leading to spiritual death (separation from God) and eventual physical death is called the 'law of sin and death' (Romans 8:2). Included in the consequences of that law are sickness, the curse that came upon the earth, human suffering and what is listed under the curse of the law (Deuteronomy 28:15-68). I need to repeat that if someone is sick it does not mean that it is because of some sin in their life. Rather this is discussing the original entry point of sickness, pain and suffering into the earth.

The law of sin and death:

immediate	←	over a period of time		→
SIN →	SPIRITUAL →	SICKNESS & DISEASE →	PHYSICAL
	DEATH	HUMAN SUFFERING	DEATH
		THE CURSE	

← root cause	→←	fruit	→

Romans 8:1, 2
There is therefore now no condemnation to those who are in Christ Jesus, who do not walk according to the flesh, but according to the Spirit. For the law of the Spirit of life in Christ Jesus has made me free from the law of sin and death.

This scripture gives us the good news. When we receive Christ, all sins committed up to that point are forgiven and removed from us, and the Holy Spirit comes and breathes the life of God into us again. We experience that spirit-to-Spirit contact that Adam once enjoyed with God. This new system of the law of the Spirit of life sets us free from the whole process of the law of sin and death. Through faith in Christ we are set free from sin, its punishment and its consequences.

All of our sin, sickness, sufferings and the curse were put on Jesus in our place and the Bible says that He actually became sin for us, that is, our sin sacrifice, in order to set us free from it.

Isaiah 53:6
And the Lord has laid on Him the iniquity of us all.

2 Corinthians 5:21
For He made Him who knew no sin to be sin for us that we might become the righteousness of God in Him.

Jesus suffered for our sin, and by association, all of the law of sin and death, which included sickness. He rose from the dead, as the life of the Holy Spirit came into His Spirit and He was 'born again', that is, He became the firstborn from the dead.

That life then affected His body and His body was resurrected an eternal, glorified body. For this reason, shouldn't we expect that when the Holy Spirit comes to give us the New Birth that His life in our spirits will work its way out to affect our physical bodies?

Romans 8:11

But if the Spirit of Him Who raised Jesus from the dead dwells in you, He Who raised Christ from the dead <u>will also give life to your mortal bodies</u> through His Spirit who dwells in you.

Galatians 3:13

Christ has redeemed us from the curse of the law, having become a curse for us...

Jesus also redeemed us from the entire curse that came upon the earth due to sin, including what is listed under the curse of the law in Deuteronomy 28:15-68. The latter includes many sicknesses and afflictions and then goes on to say in verse 61 that it also includes all the sicknesses not listed there. In addition it includes poverty, broken relationships, calamity and life not going well for you. We are not under the law but the effects of sin in the earth, which are reflected in what is described as the curse of the law (Deuteronomy 28:15-68), were experienced long before the law articulated what they were.

Under the old covenant a person experienced the effects of the curse when they were disobedient to the law. From this the curse of the law has been viewed to be the judgment of God and brought by God. However, can God bring something that is against His will, that is, sickness upon mankind?

Many believe that the verses in Deuteronomy 28 outlining the curses God will bring on disobedience are in the permissive rather than the causative case in the original Hebrew text. This means that God allowed it to happen rather than Him directly causing it. Faith in God and their obedience to Him, which included the blood sacrifices to cover their sin, protected them from the curse that was operational in the earth.

I am not a Hebrew scholar but in context with the character of God, especially in the Person of Jesus and the extraordinary lengths that He went to in order to bring us healing, it makes sense to me for God to allow the curse rather than bring it.

The earth came under a curse due to sin; that curse including the works of the devil upon mankind. 1 John 3:8 says, *'For this purpose the Son of God was manifested that he might destroy the works of the devil'.* Through the covenants, God brought to mankind a covering and protection from the curse and the works of the demonic realm. When we turn to him in faith we find protection and the works of the devil are destroyed over our lives. If we move away from His covering, that is, out of faith and obedience then we can be exposed once more to the curse. It is still operational in the earth: God has just provided a protective covering in the midst of it. If we move away, God has allowed us to be exposed to the curse but He has not brought it.

Many people say, "Well, if God is so good, why do people suffer and terrible things happen in the world?" They are the consequences of sin in the earth and not the action of God at all. However, God has provided redemption from all of these curses, in Christ, but, as with every other promise in the Bible we have to position ourselves in faith in order to be able to receive that blessing into our lives.

It is important to clarify that if someone gets sick or experiences trouble that it does not mean that they are in sin or unbelief. Sickness and trouble came into the world originally through sin and by being in the world we can be exposed to them. However, as we look to Christ in faith, we find the healing, deliverance and redemption that He has provided for us.

PICTURE

SEE YOURSELF ON THAT PATH OF GOD'S WILL AND HIS BLESSINGS

RESIST ALL DOUBT, THOUGHTS THAT ARE CONTRARY TO THE WORD OF GOD, DISCOURAGEMENT AND TEMPTATION

STAY ON THE PATH!

3

HEALING IN REDEMPTION

Jesus, in His death and resurrection, not only dealt with man's issue of sin but with the whole of the law of sin and death. He took our sins and provided us with forgiveness. He dealt with our spiritual death by reconnecting us with God and bringing the life of God into our spirits. He took the consequences or curses due to sin, redeeming us from their terrible effects. He died in our place, and while our physical bodies will one day cease because of the effects of the law of sin and death, we will have eternal life because of what Jesus did for us and be given a new immortal body at the resurrection of the dead (1 Corinthians 15:22, 52-54).

Isaiah 53 gives us an incredible insight into what Jesus accomplished for us on the Cross. Isaiah's 66 chapters are a type, or prophetic picture, of the Bible. The first 39 chapters relate to the old covenant, with 39 books later comprising the Old Testament, and the next 27 chapters to the new covenant, with 27 books being in the New Testament. At the start of the 27 chapters that are a type of the New Testament is Isaiah 40 with the prophecy about John the Baptist (verse 3-5) and at the end, in Isaiah 66, the mention of the creation of the new heavens and a new earth (verse 22).

Isaiah 53 is situated in the centre of the 27 chapters that relate to the New Testament. It is the heart of the gospel, the best revelation of the gospel of Jesus, where Isaiah is having a vision of what happened to Christ on the Cross as it is happening. Nowhere else can we find such a detailed description of what Jesus has done for us.

Some evidence that this passage is talking about Jesus is found in the following two scriptures.

John 12:37, 38

But although He had done so many signs before them, they did not believe in Him, that the word of Isaiah the prophet might be fulfilled, which he spoke:
> *"Lord, who has believed our report?*
> *And to whom has the arm of the Lord been revealed?"*

John quotes Isaiah 53:1 as relating to the ministry of Jesus.

Acts 8:30-35

So Philip ran to him (the Ethiopian eunuch) and heard him reading the prophet Isaiah, and said, "Do you understand what you are reading?"...........The place in the scripture he read was this; He was lead as a sheep to the slaughter; and as a sheep before its shearer is silent, so He opened not His mouth. In His humiliation His justice was taken away, and who will declare His generation? For His life is taken from the earth. (Isaiah 53:7-8)

So the eunuch answered Philip and said, "I ask you, of whom does the prophet say this, of himself or of some other man?" Then Philip opened his mouth, and <u>beginning at this scripture, preached Jesus to him.</u>

I'll start with Isaiah 52:13, 14. This passage is still talking about the sin-bearing servant, Jesus. Originally Scripture was not divided into chapter and verse; the translators labelled the Scriptures thus for ease of reference.

Isaiah 52; 13, 14

Behold My Servant shall deal prudently; He shall be exalted and extolled and be very high. Just as many were astonished at you, so His visage was marred more than any man, and His form more than the sons of men.

The Complete Jewish Bible puts verse 14 as, *'Just as many were appalled at him, because he was so disfigured that he didn't even seem human and simply no longer looked like a man'.*[4]

Isaiah 52:14 Amplified version
(For many the Servant of God became an object of horror; many were astonished at Him.) His face and His whole appearance were marred more than any man's, and His form beyond that of the sons of men...[3]

It goes on to say that *"just as many were astonished at Him'* so He would sprinkle the nations providing atonement for them. The different versions all seem to bring out an impact on both Jesus' appearance and form as if they are two separate things.

I believe that Isaiah is bringing out an unprecedented suffering experienced both in the spirit and the body of Jesus. Jesus bore all sin in our place, to the extent that 2 Corinthians 5:21 says that 'He became sin' for us. That just sounds blasphemous to speak of Jesus in that manner but it's really showing us the extent of abasement and suffering that He had to go to, in order to remove sin from us. The sin of one person mars them but Jesus was taking the sin of all of mankind, and so, He was marred more than any other man.

Jesus' body was then impacted with the force of sickness and disease, and of pain, that came as a consequence of the sins of mankind, and the whole of the law of sin and death that He was bearing on our behalf. You cannot sin in isolation from its consequences, and so, Jesus could not bear our sins in isolation from also bearing their consequences on our behalf.

Isaiah 53:1
Who has believed our report? And to whom has the arm of the Lord been revealed?

The arm of the Lord is the power of God and it is revealed to those who believe His report of how things are, that is, to those who are in faith.

Isaiah 53:2

For He shall grow up before Him as a tender plant, and as a root out of dry ground. He has no form or comeliness; and when we see Him, there's no beauty that we should desire Him.

Jesus came as an entrance of divine life into religious Israel (a root out of dry ground), not as a celebrated glorious person, but through very humble circumstances.

Isaiah 53:3-6

A Man of sorrows and aquainted with grief. And we hid, as it were, our faces from Him; He was despised, and we did not esteem Him.

Surely He has borne our griefs and carried our sorrows; yet we esteemed Him stricken, smitten by God, and afflicted.

But He was wounded for our transgressions, He was bruised for our iniquities; the chastisement for our peace was upon Him, and by His stripes we are healed.

All we like sheep have gone astray; We have turned, every one, to his own way; And the Lord has laid on Him the iniquity of us all.

Our translations of the Bible have been translated from Hebrew, Aramaic and Greek. Hence, it is often good to look at the original meaning of a word or passage, as some of it can be lost in translation. This is particularly so if, in the footnotes in your Bible, another meaning is given, as is the case with verse four of this passage. The word 'griefs', according to Young's Concordance, in the Hebrew is the word 'choli' and is correctly translated 'sickness, weakness or pain'[5]. The word 'sorrows' is the Hebrew word 'makob' and is correctly translated as 'pain'[5]. My quotes are from the New King James Bible and contain these corrections in the footnotes. Therefore, Isaiah 53:4 should read 'Surely He has borne our sicknesses and weaknesses and carried our pains.'

Young's Literal Translation of the Bible puts verses 4 and 5 as, *Surely our diseases he did bear, and our pains he carried; whereas we did esteem him stricken, smitten of God, and afflicted. But he was wounded because of our transgressions, he was crushed because of our iniquities; the chastisement of our peace was upon him, and with his stripes we were healed.*[6]

The Amplified version of the Bible, which brings out in parentheses the original intended meaning that was lost in translation, puts it like this;

Surely He has borne our griefs (sicknesses, weaknesses and distresses) and carried our sorrows and pains (of punishment), yet we (ignorantly) considered Him stricken, smitten, and afflicted by God (as if with leprosy).

But He was wounded for our transgressions, He was bruised for our guilt and iniquities; the chastisement (needful to obtain) peace and well-being for us was upon Him, and with the stripes (that wounded) Him we are healed and made whole.[3]

Matthew in quoting this passage from the Hebrew in Matthew 8:16,17 correctly quotes it as meaning sickness, and not grief and sorrow. He also quotes it in context with Jesus healing the sick.

Matthew 8:16,17

When evening had come they brought to Him many who were demon-possessed. And He cast out the spirits with a word, and healed all who were sick, that it might be fulfilled which was spoken by Isaiah the prophet, saying: "He Himself took our infirmities and bore our sicknesses.

All of the sick were healed in fulfilment of the prophecy that Jesus bore the sickness of all.

Many times in Scripture, we see God transfer from one to another, as with the sins of Israel being transferred to a goat that was sent away from the people, into the wilderness. We can't physically see the transfer but according to God it is done. In the same way, you might say today, "how could Jesus have borne my sins or sicknesses 2000 years ago?" Rather than try and reason out how He achieved this, understand that when God says that He has done the transfer and we identify with that, in faith, then God responds with power as if the transfer had physically taken place.

Returning to Isaiah 53:4,5, the words 'borne' and 'carried', 'nasa' and 'cabal' in the Hebrew, are the same words in verses 11 & 12, to describe Jesus' bearing our sins as our substitute.

Isaiah 53:11,12

He shall see the labour of His soul, and be satisfied. By His knowledge my righteous servant shall justify many, for He shall <u>bear</u> their iniquities. Therefore I will divide Him a portion with the great, and He shall divide the spoil with the strong, because He poured out His soul unto death, and He was numbered with the transgressors, and He <u>bore</u> the sin of many, and made intercession for the transgressors.

'Cabal' means 'to bear a load', and 'nasa', 'to carry, lift, bear up' and , included in the definition, 'to take away or carry off'. Now in Isaiah 53:11,12 these words speak of Jesus bearing our sins, which we know from the Bible as a whole He bore as our substitute, entirely removing them from us and dealing with the sin problem in its entirety. Therefore, so too in verses 4 & 5, do they speak of substitution and a total removal of sickness from us, being borne by Jesus. He carried the load of our sickness for us and took it away from us.

Isaiah 53:5 reads '*....He was bruised for our iniquities...... and by His stripes we are healed.*' The word 'stripes' is literally 'bruise' or 'blows that cut in'. Therefore, the same 'bruise' by which Jesus suffered for our sins is the same 'bruise' by which we are healed. Isaiah is bringing out that both our sins, and our sicknesses and pains, were being borne together, in the vicarious suffering of Christ.

Similarly in 1 Peter 2:24 the word stripes is more correctly translated from the Greek word 'molops' as 'a bruise, wale or wound'.

1 Peter 2:24

Who Himself bore our sins in His own body on the tree, that we, having died to sins, might live for righteousness- by whose stripes you <u>were</u> healed.

The same means by which Jesus bore our sins is the same means by which we are healed. Note that this passage is past tense because it was fulfilled on the Cross. In Isaiah 53:5 it reads *'by whose stripes you are healed'* being in the present tense, because Isaiah is having a vision of what is happening at the time of the Cross.

Many times in Scripture you see sin and sickness dealt with together because they have the same roots and, hence, the same cure. It's important to emphasise again, that this does not mean that if someone is sick, that it is because of some unrepented sin. What it means is that when sin originally entered the earth through Adam, it brought sickness with it, and it has been present ever since. God always deals with the root cause of a problem and not just the symptoms.

I'll digress for a moment on this point. In John 9:2, having seen a man blind from birth, Jesus' disciples ask Him, *"Rabbi, who sinned, this man or his parents, that he was born blind?"* How many believers who have struggled with illness have felt the condemnation of religious thinking, or even beliefs of other religions, that their suffering or disability must be due to something they have done, or that they mustn't be doing something right. Jesus' response is, *"neither this man nor his parents sinned, but that the works of God should be revealed in him."*

Most of the time, sickness or disability is not due to the individual's sin, nor that of their parents, but the result of living in a fallen world, where sickness is present, with imperfect bodies. However, this positions them so that the works of God can be done in them and they can be healed. Note, God does not bring the sickness in order to display His healing- He is not the Author of sickness, but if it is present, as the Author of healing, He will heal the sick person.

There are a few occasions where sickness is due to the sin of the person, a couple of examples of which we will look at from the scriptures later on, but this is not the case in the majority of sicknesses. Now, we will return to Isaiah 53.

Isaiah 53:10
Yet it pleased the Lord to bruise Him; He has put Him to grief (literally sickness) *when You made His soul an offering for sin.*

Young's Literal Translation reads, '*Yet it pleased the LORD to crush him by disease; to see if his soul would offer itself in restitution, that he might see his seed, prolong his days, and that the purpose of the LORD might prosper by his hand:* '[6]

The Amplified version reads, "*Yet it was the will of the Lord to bruise Him; He has put Him to grief and made Him sick. When You and He made His life an offering for sin (and He has risen from the dead, in time to come), He shall see His (spiritual) offspring, He shall prolong His days, and the will and pleasure of the Lord shall prosper in His hands.*"[3]

It pleased God for the bruise and sickness to be placed upon Jesus because it meant that we could be completely redeemed from it, and it happened when He was being made an offering for sin. They occurred at the same time.

Now what do we understand by the word 'bruise'? If someone were to hit another person with a bat (please don't try this at home), a bruise would develop as a direct result of being hit with the bat. Well, as a result of being hit with the full force of sin, Jesus body was bruised with sickness and disease.

Jesus put an axe to the root of sickness, thereby removing the fruit of physical sickness, before it had time to manifest in His body in the six hours that He was on the Cross. For this reason, the disciples did not see His body covered with evidence of sicknesses, but He bore them just the same. He cursed sickness at its root.

Recall in Mark 11 when Jesus cursed the fig tree. He sees a fig tree with leaves, which meant that it should also have fruit. When He sees it has no fruit, He curses it and travels on into Jerusalem. That night He returns to Bethany with His disciples, past the tree but no one notices any change in it. The following morning, they return to Jerusalem, past the tree and Peter sees that it has dried up from the roots. The tree died at the instant that Jesus cursed it, but it took time for what had happened in the spirit realm to be manifested in the natural realm. In the same way, Jesus cursed sickness at the root, before it had a chance to manifest as physical sickness in His body.

Some people see the physical lashes that Jesus received as somehow transferring sickness to Him at that point. I believe that in Isaiah 53:5, *'by His stripes we are healed'* does not refer to the physical stripes or lashes that Jesus received from the Roman soldiers, but to the blows His body received as it was lashed with the full force of sickness, disease and pain in the spiritual realm.

Throughout Scripture, God gives us physical pictures of what happens in the spiritual realm to aid our understanding. For example, sowing seed and reaping harvests to instruct us about what happens when we put the Word of God into our hearts (Mark 4) or the giving of finance.

I believe that the stripes that Jesus received from the Roman soldiers, as horrific as they were, were giving us a picture of a far greater impact or bruise on His body in the realm of the spirit, as His body was lashed with our sicknesses, diseases and pains.

PICTURE

ALL OF YOUR SICKNESSES AND PAINS WERE PLACED UPON JESUS.

HE HAS SUFFERED THEM IN YOUR PLACE.

YOU ARE HEALED FROM ALL SICKNESS!

4

THE TYPE OF THE
BRAZEN SERPENT

....

A picture of the redemption that is ours in Christ is found in the story of the brazen serpent in Numbers 21. This story provides a type of our salvation and how we receive it; a type being a prophetic picture given beforehand through a person or event, of an event in the New Testament, particularly of Jesus and what He did for us.

Numbers 21:4-9

Then they journeyed from Mount Hor by the Way of the Red Sea, to go around the land of Edom; and the soul of the people became very discouraged on the way. And the people spoke against God and against Moses: "Why have you brought us up out of Egypt to die in the wilderness? For there is no food and no water, and our soul loathes this worthless bread." So the LORD sent fiery serpents among the people, and they bit the people; and many of the people of Israel died.

Therefore the people came to Moses, and said, "We have sinned, for we have spoken against the LORD and against you; pray to the LORD that He take away the serpents from us." So Moses prayed for the people.

Then the LORD said to Moses, "Make a fiery serpent, and set it on a pole; and it shall be that everyone who is bitten, when he looks at it, shall live." So Moses made a bronze serpent, and put it on a pole; and so it was, if a serpent had bitten anyone, when he looked at the bronze serpent, he lived.

According to many Bible teachers, verse six can be interpreted in the Hebrew permissive case (i.e. God allowing it) or the causative case (i.e. God causing it). While you can't be dogmatic about which one it is, the context appears to be God allowing a judgment that was of a demonic source. The judgment is God's will, but comes about as the people, by their own actions, move outside the realm of God's protection, that is, off His path of blessing, and are exposed to the work of the enemy. Note that God immediately provides a way of deliverance and healing for those who will take it.

I see the protection of God like a covering or umbrella that extends over His path for us, that is, His will. Beyond that path is where Satan can operate and where the curse due to sin in the earth can take effect. We access God's blessings, including redemption from the effects of sin and protection from the works of darkness, by faith and obedience. If we are not in that position of faith and obedience, God doesn't come running after us with His umbrella to cover us in our unbelief or disobedience. We have to position ourselves on God's path in order to enjoy all that Jesus has purchased for us.

The Hebrews moved away from God and His protection, through unbelief (Hebrews 3:12) and disobedience. They were then exposed to the consequences for sin and the works of darkness. Repentance and faith in God's means of deliverance brought them back under the umbrella of His protection.

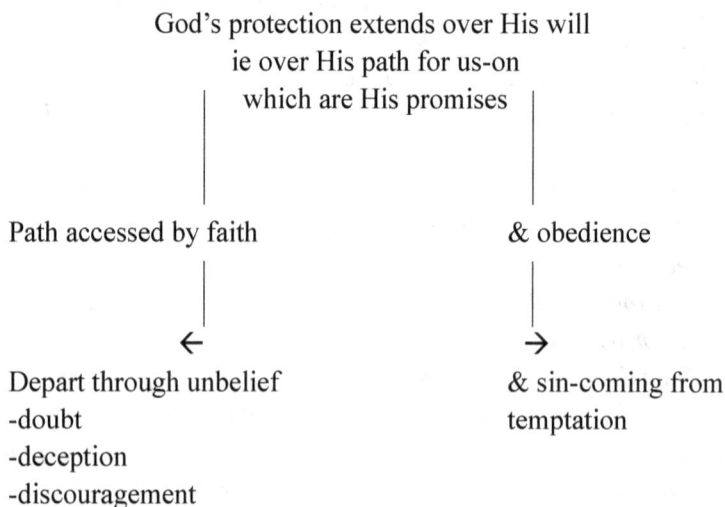

God's protection extends over His will
ie over His path for us-on
which are His promises

Path accessed by faith   & obedience

←   →

Depart through unbelief   & sin-coming from
-doubt   temptation
-deception
-discouragement

Looking at Numbers 21:4, *'and the soul of the people became very discouraged on the way'* and 21:5, *"Why have you brought us up out of Egypt to die in the wilderness?"* They were in unbelief and discouragement, and not in faith. Faith in God and His word involves believing the truth in your heart, speaking (or confessing) that truth to release your faith and, then, acting on that truth. Or, more likely, you find that your actions naturally follow what you believe and speak. Unbelief or fear operates in the negative realm in exactly the same way, believing that something negative will happen, speaking it out of your mouth and then your actions or circumstances naturally follow.

God's continual problem with the children of Israel was their unbelief and negative heart attitudes, which led to negative speaking, murmuring and grumbling and then to sin and rebellion. Their actions then put them in a place outside of God's covering and protection.

Hebrews 3:12,13
Beware, brethren, lest there be in any of you an evil heart of unbelief in departing from the living God; but exhort one another daily, while it is called "Today", lest any of you be hardened through the deceitfulness of sin.

Unbelief causes you to depart from that place under God's covering. It's a challenge for all of us that God calls it evil to believe the negative report instead of His word. Unbelief deceives us that there is another truth, other than God's and leads to sin, which in turn, hardens our heart. Unbelief lies at the root of all disobedience, just as faith lies at the root of obedience.

Hebrews 3:16-19
For who, having heard, rebelled? Indeed, was it not all who came out of Egypt, led by Moses? Now with whom was He angry forty years? Was it not with those who sinned, whose corpses fell in the wilderness? And to whom did He swear that they would not enter His rest, but to those who did not obey? So we see that they could not enter in because of unbelief.

Note that the heart attitude of unbelief in verse 12 led to the sin and disobedience in verses 16-19. For this reason they could not enter God's blessings, and for the same reason, that is, unbelief, we can depart from His blessing and protection.

Back in Numbers 21, the people of God are dying from poisonous snake bites. They repent of their sin, their grumbling and rebellious attitudes reflected in calling God's provision 'this worthless bread', and appeal to Moses to pray for them. The Lord gives Moses instructions to make a bronze serpent and set it up on a pole so that everyone could look upon it. Those who looked at the bronze serpent lived and, therefore, they must have been healed of their bites and delivered from the serpents that were still round them.

The serpent on a pole was a type of Jesus on the Cross, as Jesus explains in John 3:14-16.

John 3:14-16

And as Moses lifted up the serpent in the wilderness, even so must the Son of Man be lifted up, that whoever believes in Him should not perish but have eternal life. For God so loved the world that He gave His only begotten Son, that whoever believes in Him should not perish but have everlasting life.

In Numbers 21, it was through faith in a type of Jesus on the Cross, that the serpent which caused the affliction was removed, and the people were healed.

It is an interesting analogy of the serpent on a pole representing Jesus. John the Baptist referred to Jesus as *'the Lamb of God who takes away the sin of the world'* (John 1:29) and, yet, we see a serpent and not a lamb in this type. The serpent, in the Bible, represents the devil, the source of sin and death, and his power.

Genesis 3:1

Now the serpent was more cunning than any beast of the field which the Lord God had made.

Luke 10:19

Behold, I give you authority to trample on serpents and scorpions, and over all the power of the enemy, and nothing shall by any means hurt you.

Rev 20:2

He laid hold of the dragon, that serpent of old, who is the devil and Satan...

Now it was a serpent on that pole because Jesus, the spotless Lamb of God, became the sacrifice for sin and sickness for us, in order to give us life. In removing our sin, He also removed the devil's power over mankind that had its entry point through sin. The serpent was a picture of what Jesus was bearing and destroying the power of, for us, and not a picture of He Himself.

2 Corinthians 5:21

For He made Him who knew no sin to be sin for us, that we might become the righteousness of God in Him.

Isaiah 53:6

And the Lord has laid on Him the iniquity of us all.

Galatians 3:13 says that, *'Christ has redeemed us from the curse of the law, having become a curse for us'*. Not only did Jesus become sin for us, that is, our sacrifice for sin, He also became the curse for us. He bore the curse that included sickness and the works of the devil on our behalf, setting us free from it.

The serpents, their bite and poison are types of Satan and his power, sin that allows his power to enter, and its consequences. So, when Jesus took our sin to the Cross, He also took Satan's power over us and nailed it there too.

1 John 3:8

For this purpose the Son of God was manifested, that He might destroy the works of the devil.

Colossians 1:13, 14 (speaking of Jesus)

He has delivered us from the power of darkness and conveyed us into the kingdom of the Son of His love, in whom we have redemption through His blood, the forgiveness of sins. (It's past tense because it happened on the Cross).

Colossians 2:15

Having disarmed (stripped of power and authority) principalities and powers, He made a public spectacle of them, triumphing over them in it ('it' being the Cross).

Hebrews 2:14 Amplified

...that by (going through) death He might bring to nought and make of no effect him who had the power of death – that is, the devil.[3]

In the Garden of Eden, God cursed the serpent, the devil saying "I will put enmity between you and the woman and between your seed and her Seed; He shall bruise your head and you shall bruise His heel" (Genesis 3:15).

Note that He did not curse Adam and Eve. He cursed the ground that Adam worked on, which I believe is a picture of the works of the flesh or our own efforts, and He cursed the devil. This is a type of what Jesus would fulfil for us. In Him, works of the flesh are cursed and won't achieve the purposes of God, and so too, is the devil cursed.

The seed of the woman is Jesus. We are said to be born of the seed of a man but Jesus was born of the seed of woman because He was born of a virgin. God promised that Christ would bruise the devil's head, which is his power or authority, but in the process He would be bruised. The bruising of the heel took place when Jesus died on the Cross. When a person is crucified, they push themself up by the heel to get more air into the lungs, thereby bruising their heel.

Satan bruised the heel of the seed of the woman, but, seeing a physical picture of what was happening spiritually, as the devil struck His heel, Jesus brought down His foot and crushed the devil's head, thus crushing his power and authority.

The devil had thought that he had Jesus defeated but he did not know what God had in mind. By the same process where he thought he was striking down Jesus, his power and authority was stripped from him.

1 Corinthians 2:7, 8

But we speak the wisdom of God in a mystery, the hidden wisdom which God ordained before the ages for our glory, which none of the rulers of this age knew; for had they known, they would not have crucified the Lord of glory.

Returning to Numbers 21, any person who 'looked at' the brazen serpent lived, was delivered from the serpents and was healed. See the picture of Christ on the Cross! It was not the serpent on the pole that healed them but faith in God that He would heal them as they obeyed His Word and looked to the vision of what Christ would do for us. In fact, later on, the Israelites make the mistake of worshipping the method, that is, the bronze serpent, rather than the God Who employed the method. In 2 Kings 18:4, Hezekiah destroys the bronze serpent because the children of Israel had made an idol of it.

The Amplified Bible interpretation for *'looked at'* is to *'look attentively, expectantly, and with a steady and absorbing gaze'*[3]. If we look at something attentively, it means that it has all of our focus; we are looking at it carefully, noting every detail. To look at it expectantly implies that we are expecting something to happen in response to that look and so, it is talking about the look of faith. To look with a steady and absorbing gaze means that we not only keep looking at it, as opposed to a mere glance, but we are absorbing something from it. Therefore, we are influenced and are changed by what we are looking at.

It's good to note that the Israelites couldn't look at the bronze snake and their symptoms at the same time. Paul writes in Romans 4 that Abraham's faith grew strong while he looked at the promise of God. Some people reverse this and their faith grows weak while they look at their symptoms and forget the promise.

James 1:22-25 NIV

Do not merely listen to the word, and so deceive yourselves. Do what it says.

Anyone who listens to the word but does not do what it says is like a man who looks at his face in a mirror and, after looking at himself, goes away and immediately forgets what he looks like.

But the man who looks intently into the perfect law that gives freedom, and continues to do this, not forgetting what he has heard but doing it – he will be blessed in what he does.[7]

As we look into God's Word we see who we really are, the self created in His image. The person we see in His Word is already healed 'by the stripes of Jesus'. If we do not attend to this truth, continually looking into the mirror of the Word, then we go away and forget that we have been healed and we see the symptoms of sickness instead. If we only hear the truth about healing but don't attend to it, looking intently into it, we fail to appropriate that truth in our life and end up seeing sickness rather than healing, thus deceiving ourselves that we are not a healed person.

We need to be looking intently and continually into the word of God. If it's healing that we need, then we need to be looking intently and continuously at Scriptures on healing. We are to look attentively, absorbingly, being changed by what we are looking at, and expectantly bringing faith, which empowers us to obey and positions us receive the promise.

The Lord showed me that it is not enough to just memorise the Scriptures any more than it was enough for the Israelites to just remember what the serpent on a pole looked like. We have to be continually looking at the Scriptures until healed. The healing process goes on while we are looking at the promise.

2 Corinthians 3:18

But we all, with unveiled face, beholding as in a mirror the glory of the Lord, are being transformed into the same image from glory to glory, just as by the Spirit of the Lord.

Paul, like James, likens the word of God to a mirror that we look into, but the image we see is Jesus Himself; Jesus, who bore our sins and carried our sicknesses and *'by whose stripes we are healed'*. The analogy is that, as we look intently into the word of God, we are looking intently at the image of Jesus. In the same way, the Israelites looked intently at the type of Jesus in the form of the brazen serpent, being attentive to the image of Him, influenced by what they saw and expectant to receive and were healed. Now, if they received healing and deliverance through faith in a type of Christ on the Cross, how much more shall we receive healing and deliverance through faith in Jesus Himself.

PICTURE

JESUS ON THE CROSS BEARING ALL YOUR SIN, SICKNESS AND ALL THE POWER OF THE DEVIL

KEEP LOOKING AT HIM, THROUGH HIS WORD, UNTIL HEALED!

5

RECEIVING HEALING BY FAITH

....

HEALING AND FORGIVENESS
ARE PROVIDED TOGETHER

One day I was talking to a lady who was a counsellor and she said to me, "it is more important for someone to be forgiven and at peace in their emotions than it is to have physical healing." If you had to make a choice between them, I would have to agree with her, but the fact is you don't have to choose because they all come together in the one salvation- Jesus covered it all.

Ephesians 2:8, 9
For by grace you have been saved through faith and that not of yourselves; it is the gift of God, not of works lest anyone should boast.

The word translated salvation here is the Greek word 'sozo' which, according to Strong's Concordance, means 'to save, that is, deliver, or protect (figuratively and literally); heal, preserve, do well, be or make whole'[2]. Our English word 'salvation' does not adequately describe all that the Greek word 'sozo' encompasses.

Salvation is a package deal. You put your faith in Christ's sacrifice and healing comes as well as forgiveness, deliverance and eternal life. When you see the word saved in Scripture, you can also insert healed. Sometimes the word 'sozo' is used for healing, and sometimes for eternal life – both are encompassed in the one word. Forgiveness of sin and healing are combined together throughout Scripture.

The following are a few examples of the use of the word 'sozo' in the gospels. The woman with the issue of blood (a physical problem) being healed is recorded in Matthew 9:18-22. In **Matthew 9:22**, Jesus says ' *Be of good cheer daughter; your faith has made you well.* ' 'Well' is translated from '*sozo*'.

In **Mark 6:56**, *Wherever He (Jesus) entered, into villages, cities, or the country, they laid the sick in the market places, and begged Him that they might just touch the hem of His garment. And as many as touched Him were made well.* Once again '*sozo*' is translated as 'well'.

Mark 10:46-52 is the healing of blind Bartimaeus.

Mark 10:52
Then Jesus said to him "Go your way, your faith has made you well" (sozo) And immediately he received his sight and followed Jesus on the road.

Luke 17:12-19 records the healing of the 10 lepers with one returning to thank Jesus. In verse 19, Jesus said to him "*Arise, go your way; your faith has made you well.*" 'Well' is translated from '*sozo*'. The Amplified version says '*your faith (your trust and confidence that spring from your belief in God) has restored you to health.* '[3]

It could be that all ten were healed of the leprosy but this one was restored to wholeness, that is to say, that the parts of the flesh that had been eaten away were restored, or it could be that this man received eternal life as well as his healing. The Message Bible says "*your faith has healed and saved you*".[8]

In all of these Scriptures it is a physical sickness that is being healed. In the following scriptures the word 'sozo' is translated as saved, meaning forgiveness of sins and eternal salvation.

Acts 16:31

Believe on the Lord Jesus Christ, and you will be saved, you and your household. 'Saved' is translated from *'sozo'.*

Acts 4:12

Nor is there salvation in any other, for there is no other name under heaven given among men by which we must be saved. 'Saved' is translated from *'sozo'.*

Romans 10:13

For "whoever calls upon the name of the Lord shall be saved" 'Saved' is translated from *'sozo'.*

So the word used for eternal salvation and forgiveness of sin is exactly the same as that for being healed. God has provided for every part of our being and every part of our lives with His salvation. Salvation is not just for our spirit, but our spirit, soul and body.

1 Thessalonians 5:23

Now may the God of peace Himself sanctify you completely; and may your whole spirit, soul and body be preserved blameless at the coming of our Lord Jesus Christ.

Matthew 9:2-8, Mark 2:3-12 and Luke 5:18-26 record the healing of the paralytic, whose four friends carried him and let him down through the roof of the house where Jesus was preaching.

Matthew 9:2

Then behold, they brought to Him a paralytic lying on a bed. When Jesus saw their faith, He said to the paralytic, "Son, be of good cheer; your sins are forgiven you."

Matthew 9:5-7

For which is easier, to say, 'Your sins are forgiven you,' or to say, 'Arise and walk'? But that you may know that the Son of Man has power on earth to forgive sins"—then He said to the paralytic, "Arise, take up your bed, and go to your house." And he arose and departed to his house.

Jesus was saying that for Him to say the man was forgiven was the same as for Him to say that He was healed. They are both part of His salvation for mankind and can't be separated. As far as God is concerned if you are forgiven, then you are healed- we just have to receive it.

With that in mind, look at Ephesians 2:8, *'For by grace you have been saved* (delivered, protected, healed, preserved, made well, made whole) *through faith'*.

By grace you <u>have been healed</u>, made whole through faith. It's past tense!

So often when we pray for healing, we plead with God or try to persuade Him to heal us. As far as God is concerned, He has already healed us, just as He has already forgiven us. He looks back on the Cross of Calvary and sees all of your sicknesses, as well as your sins, placed upon Jesus. All of His promises are already provided through the sacrifice of Jesus. All the promises of God are 'yes and amen' in Him (2 Corinthians 1:20).

It only needs, now, for us to receive what He has already freely given us by His grace. Now, in order to receive from God, we have to get in agreement with Him and see our healing as being already provided for us, despite how we are feeling and the symptoms that are still present in our body, before that healing manifests physically.

Before we go on to the next chapter on how to receive healing, it might be a good place to answer the question that arises every time I take a healing course. So many people ask, "what about so and so who prayed and believed and wasn't healed"; "what if someone doesn't get healed"; "if God has already healed us, then why do some faithful Christians die prematurely?"

I don't have the answers to all the questions people have, but all I can do is share what the Lord said to me on one occasion. As a group of believers, we had been praying for another leader who was suffering a terminal illness. Everyone was believing God and yet this person died. Knowing the Lord to be our Healer, I went to Him and asked, "Well, what was all that about?"

He promptly answered me, "Run with what you know, not with what you don't know." So, what do I know? I know that God is Who He says He is and has done what He has said He has done, whether it manifests in my life or the life of another, or not. He is the Healer. Jesus has born our sicknesses and carried our pains. He heals all our diseases.

What I don't know is why that believer died. However, we have to run with what we do know, not with what we don't know. We only know in part and see in a mirror dimly (1 Corinthians 13:12). We see a tiny part of the picture, and even that, not too clearly. Only God knows the whole picture.

However if we get stuck on the times when things don't go the way that we believed, then we won't stay in faith and we won't get moving again in reaching out to people with God's healing grace. We won't be able to either believe for healing for ourselves or minister healing to another who needs it. The fact is, when we position ourselves in faith the way that I am about to share with you, healing will manifest the majority of times.

PICTURE

SEE YOURSELF AS ALREADY HAVING HEALING PROVIDED FOR YOU JUST AS FORGIVENESS OF SIN HAS ALREADY BEEN PROVIDED.

GOD SEES YOU HEALED

CHOOSE TO SEE YOUSELF THE SAME WAY

KEYS TO POSITIONING YOURSELF
TO RECEIVE HEALING

I am going to take you through the process the Lord showed me, to position yourself to receive your healing. It is important to keep in mind that you are healed by grace and that you receive it through faith. Too many people confuse this as being 'I am healed by faith', 'If I just have enough faith, if I just speak the Word enough, if I'm just good enough at this, then I will be healed'. Don't get me wrong, we do need faith and we do need to speak God's Word but it's not your faith that heals you. There is nothing you can do to make your healing available to you and nothing that you can do to earn it. Jesus has already done this for you.

Faith simply positions you to receive what He has already provided for you. Jesus said that if you have faith the size of a tiny mustard seed it has the potential to bring about something great. We need to understand that it's not about us and how great our faith is; it's all about Jesus and how great He is in all that He has already done for us.

There are also those I have ministered to, who were either sick, even with a terminal illness, or were unable to have children, who have disputed that they don't need to do the process of faith that I am about to outline to you. Many Christians feel that they don't need to follow the way of faith or have to be in the Word of God, believing for their healing. Many want to do it 'their own way'. Since it is the Bible that is directing us to this path of faith in order to receive from God, and since those that are waiting for another way rarely get healed, I am not convinced by their arguments.

Others have said, "Well, God knows I am having a hard time. He should meet me where I'm at". I have found that unless you are a new believer or new to teaching on faith and healing or, unless you are too unwell to read the Bible or pray, then God doesn't seem to meet us where we are at. He wants us to meet Him where He's at, and for us that is a place of faith in Him and His Word.

Too many Christians want the easy path to healing. As a pastor, they want you to keep laying hands on them, keep praying for them, keep visiting them until they are healed. Or, they are waiting for a healing ministry to come to church so that they can be healed on the altar call at the end of the message.

Don't misunderstand me, many people are healed through such ministry which is wonderful, and many are healed when we pray for them. However, since so many of the healings in the Bible, particularly Jesus' ministry, were attributed to the faith of the person being healed, this tells me that faith is an integral part of receiving God's healing power at least some of the time, but really I would suggest, most of the time.

God doesn't want us to always be waiting for someone else to do the believing, praying and delving into the Word for us. He wants us to be that person! There may be times when we will need that prayer from a pastor or healing minister but this should not be the mainstay of our receiving from God. He wants us to be that person who can not only receive directly from Him, through His Word and the ministry of the Holy Spirit, but who can also be the one to minister to others.

It is also good to be aware that after receiving the healing anointing after prayer at the altar, this deposit of God's power still needs to be worked out, through standing in faith. Don't be discouraged if you are not instantly healed at times of prayer by an anointed minister. God's healing power has been deposited in you and, as you walk in faith, that healing power will have its effect in your physical body.

In the same way, healings that are received through anointed prayer, are sometimes lost, the healing deteriorating over time. Faith is required to maintain the healing that has been received through prayer or anointed ministry.

BELIEVE GOD AND
ATTEND TO HIS WORD

Particularly when you are facing a major illness, or indeed any difficult situation, your circumstances and the facts of those circumstances do not look remotely like that which the Bible is declaring. We have to make a choice to believe God and then to trust Him that He and the power of His Word are more than enough to change the facts of our circumstances.

Proverbs 4:20-27 provides a pattern for us, that I will draw upon over the four steps that I will discuss in receiving healing. When I speak of steps, it is with the intention of providing a clear pattern of how to receive from God and is in no way intended to be some formula that we mechanically put into practice, apart from a living relationship with Him.

Proverbs 4:20-27
My son, give attention to my words;
Incline your ear to my sayings.
Do not let them depart from your eyes;
Keep them in the midst of your heart;
For they are life to those who find them,
And health to all their flesh.
Keep your heart with all diligence,
For out of it spring the issues of life.
Put away from you a deceitful mouth,
And put perverse lips far from you.
Let your eyes look straight ahead,

And your eyelids look right before you.
Ponder the path of your feet,
And let all your ways be established.
Do not turn to the right or the left;
Remove your foot from evil.

Starting with the first line, '*My son, give attention to my words*'. I found that this has to be a conscious decision because there are many words out there and few of them are positive when you are facing a serious or impossible situation. To attend to something is to give all of your focus to it; your mind is directed to it; you are 'in the moment', that is, carefully thinking on that thing whilst blocking out all distractions.

I found that I had to continually attend to the Word of God to contend with all the contrary words and reports that would come my way. The Lord, on one such occasion, showed me a valuable insight on this. When I was struggling with serious illness and 'trying to believe' in the early days, well- meaning people would call me up regularly, saying 'I know what you are facing; I know how sick you are; you are not facing reality thinking that you will be healed.'

As I cried out to God, He directed me to Romans 3:3, 4.

Romans 3:3,4

For what if some did not believe? Will their unbelief make the faithfulness of God without effect? Certainly not! Indeed, let God be true but every man a liar. As it is written: "That You may be justified in your words, and may overcome when You are judged".

The NIV in verse 3 says, '*What if some did not have faith? Will their lack of faith nullify God's faithfulness?*' The Lord spoke to me and said, "It doesn't matter what they believe Kate; it matters what you believe." Someone else's lack of faith or negative words can't stop you being healed. The devil's lies and bombardment of negativity and doubt against your mind can't stop you being healed. The only way they can hinder you receiving your healing is if you choose to give attention to their words instead of God's.

Paul declares to us in Romans 3:4, to let God and His words be our truth, and those that declare otherwise to be liars (even though it be unconsciously so in them). He then states that God's Word will be declared to be right and true and will overcome no matter who challenges it. Proverbs 2:12 says that God overthrows the words of the faithless.

Another thing that the Lord said to me was, 'listen to Me and you will live'. He then started to direct me to all these scriptures, as well as Proverbs 4:20-22, on how keeping God's Word brings life.

Proverbs 3:1
....But let your heart keep my commands; For length of days and long life and peace they will add to you.

Proverbs 4:4
...let your heart retain my words; keep my commands and live.

Proverbs 9:11
For by me your days will be multiplied, and years of life will be added to you.

Proverbs 10:27
The fear of the Lord prolongs days...

We need to attend to what the Lord is saying to us in His Word and by the Holy Spirit, more than the words of others, even those who are experts in the facts. This does not mean that we don't go to doctors, respect and follow their advice or reject medication if it's needed. It is wisdom to seek medical advice when facing serious illness and medication is often life-saving. It just means that we need to attend to God's Word over and above that of others.

It is often a great testimony to the medical profession when people have been under their care and then, they are miraculously healed. My husband, Richard, and I were called to pray for a lady one day, who had been given 24 hours to live. She had Lymphoma with resultant major organ problems, a bleeding duodenal ulcer and kidney failure. Of course, many others were praying for her healing, but we had the privilege to lay hands on her in the name of Jesus and pray that her healing be released. That beautiful lady was out of hospital within 2 weeks and back at work 5 days after that, with no evidence of any cancer and with her kidney function restored. This is a great testimony to doctors, who had told the family that 'it would not be long now'.

Jesus indicates in Matthew 8:4, following the cleansing of the leper, that it's alright to get the clearance from the doctor that the sickness is dealt with (that clearance coming from the priests in His time on earth), which means that for those with serious illness, they needed to be under medical care in the first place. This clearance then becomes a testimony to the medical practitioner.

Matthew 8:4
And Jesus said to him, "See that you tell no one; but go your way, show yourself to the priest, and offer the gift that Moses commanded, as a testimony to them."

My thoughts are that medical advice should be sought for serious illness and treatment followed, whilst believing God all the time for His healing and complete recovery. Often healing is a process or it takes time also for us to figure out how to receive it, especially initially, and it's good to be under medical wisdom while waiting for your healing to manifest. Their word is just not the final word- God's Word is!

To say that it is unbelieving to seek medical advice is like saying that because we trust God for financial provision, then we should never get financial advice nor see accountants or investment experts, because theirs is just worldly wisdom. That is just foolishness! Of course we seek advice from those trained in their areas of expertise and we operate in wisdom as well as faith. However, while operating in wisdom and common sense, we put, above all else, our faith in God who is our Healer.

As an aside, personally, I am very cautious about the seeking of many of the alternate therapies. Too many of them have a spiritual side to them that is not of God. You can take it or leave it, but I have noted that those who follow after many of the alternate therapies seem to have a 'veil' over their spiritual eyes regarding God's healing and not only don't see it, but don't receive it. I don't know whether this is solely spiritual or also because too many people see certain therapies, diets, or special preparations as being their source of healing, and their eyes are not on Jesus.

We do need to 'work with' God and be wise in how we take care of our bodies by eating well, avoiding putting toxins or any causes of sickness into our bodies, and exercising. They just don't become our 'god' or source. It's no use eating rubbish, and not exercising and then expecting God to heal your blood pressure when it goes up. It's no use to be a chain smoker and then ask God to protect you from lung cancer. God will still heal you as you make the necessary lifestyle adjustments, but if He healed you without you making the lifestyle changes, your body would just head back to that sickness again.

Another problem that many believers deal with is the unbelief of ministers or others to whom they have gone for advice, or religious traditions. I have often had the opportunity to pray for people for healing who have not been able to have this prayer in their own churches.

It amazes me the teaching given to so many today which contradicts the Bible and the practices of Jesus, the disciples and the believers of the early church. Some are told that God no longer heals, that only the original 12 apostles had the gift of healing, that God put sickness on them to teach them something, that God uses sickness to bring about good in their lives or the lives of others. Others are told that 'your suffering is bringing glory to Him', that the healing in the early church came through a special oil used in those days that we no longer have available and that sometimes, the answer is just 'no'.

To my mind, many of the erroneous teachings that have arisen in the church (erroneous because they contradict God and His Word) have come about because healings have not occurred or God has not moved in a way that was prayed for. So, rather than looking to themselves and seeing where they needed to change, too many people have blamed God for changing His character or His ways.

Hebrew 13:8 tells us that Jesus, our Healer, is the same yesterday, today and forever. Forever is He our Healer. For healing to have passed away, salvation would have had to pass away as they are part of the same package. At no point in Jesus' ministry does He say 'no' to anyone seeking healing. Some cite the story in Matthew 15:21-28 of the Syro-Phoenician woman whose daughter has a demonic spirit. Jesus, I believe, delays the release of the healing in order to draw out of her the evidence of a faith that He wanted to display to others, but He does heal her daughter.

God will not put sickness on you to teach you something. At no point in Jesus' ministry does He put sickness on anyone. God is Jehovah Rapha, the 'Lord who heals'; it's not just what He does but who He is.

Matthew 7:11
If you then, being evil, know how to give good gifts to your children, how much more will your Father who is in heaven give good things to those who ask Him.

The Bible is not saying we are evil people, but in comparison to the extreme goodness of God, we would be. Now, we wouldn't put cancer on our children in order to teach them something and yet, God, who is Love, full of mercy and loving kindness, is often accused of doing just that. God corrects us with His Word in the same way that we would do with our children.

2 Timothy 3:16
All Scripture is given by inspiration of God, and is profitable for doctrine, for reproof, for correction, for instruction in righteousness,

Some people believe, falsely, that God not only teaches us through sickness but He uses it for His glory. One day I had a lady come to me with what she thought was a great testimony. It went like this. She had broken her leg in a car accident and, while in hospital, was able to witness about Christ to the lady in the bed next to her. She concluded, based on Romans 8:28, which many use in such cases, that God was so good to bring the accident as it enabled the gospel to come to that lady.

Romans 8:28

And we know that all things work together for good to those who love God, to those who are the called according to His purpose.

Romans 8:28 is in context with intercessory prayer. When we don't know what to pray for, the Holy Spirit will pray through us, using the gift of tongues, the perfect will of God for that situation, thus allowing God to move in that situation. He will then work all things together for your good. It isn't saying that God will bring evil, sickness or accidents to use them for some assumed purpose.

God gets no glory from people suffering, nor would He seek such. Throughout the gospels, people glorified God when they saw the sick being healed, not for seeing people suffering. To say that God gets glory from your suffering would be like saying that God gets glory from your sin, seeing that He has considered them to be part of the same law. Sin and sickness are so abhorrent to Him that He suffered unbelievably in order to set us free from them.

Matthew 15:30,31

Then great multitudes came to Him, having with them the lame, blind, mute, maimed, and many others; and they laid them down at Jesus' feet, and He healed them. So the multitude marveled when they saw the mute speaking, the maimed made whole, the lame walking, and the blind seeing; and they glorified the God of Israel.

The other area of unbelief is that some falsely believe that only Jesus or only the twelve disciples had the power to heal the sick. We will look at, in more detail, the power that Jesus intends for all believers to operate in, later on in 'The commission to heal the sick'. In the meantime, I will just add in the following scripture where Jesus Himself states His intention for all to do His works.

John 14:12
Most assuredly, I say to you, <u>he who believes in Me</u>, <u>the works that I do he will do also</u>; and <u>greater works than these he will do</u>, because I go to My Father.

These teachings place people in a state of unbelief, thereby, preventing them from receiving from God. Even Jesus, being God Himself and having the Holy Spirit without measure, could do not mighty miracles in His home town of Nazareth because of their unbelief. God has set things up so that we receive His grace, and thereby all of His promises which are given by grace, through our faith. Unbelief stops you receiving God's grace and promises.

In Mark 9 and Matthew 17 is the story of an epileptic boy, who is suffering from a demonic spirit, and the disciples find they can't cast it out. In the latter part of Mark 9:22, the boy's father says to Jesus, "But if you can do anything, have compassion on us and help us". Jesus is very quick to respond in the following scripture; it's not whether He can do anything but it's whether we can believe.

Mark 9:24
Jesus said to him, "If you can believe, all things are possible to him who believes."

In Matthew 17:20, Jesus also rebukes His disciples for their unbelief. In Matthew 10:1, Jesus had commissioned them, giving them 'power over unclean spirits to cast them out, and to heal all kinds of sickness and all kinds of disease'. They should have been able to cast the spirit out but unbelief limited them. Later on Jesus tells them that this kind only comes out by prayer and fasting which many take to mean that they couldn't have cast this one out anyway because it was particularly difficult.

I don't see that as the case. Jesus hadn't commissioned them to cast out all spirits except the difficult ones. He gave them authority over all the power of the enemy (Luke 10:17). They should have been able to do it. However, unbelief lowers the level of the anointing that a person operates in, which we will look at later on in 'Ministering healing". When the anointing level drops, I have found that prayer and fasting, as well as increased attention to the Word, is required to get it back.

In Mark 5, Jesus is coming to the house of the one of the rulers of the synagogue because his daughter is very ill and in fact, Jesus will need to raise her from the dead. The man believes that Jesus will heal her, evidenced in verse 23, "My little daughter lies at the point of death. Come and lay your hands on her, that she may be healed, and she will live."

Soon after, some from his household come and say that she is dead and not to bother Jesus any longer. The temptation to get off the track of believing, through fear, doubt or discouragement has come, and Jesus moves immediately to make sure that the man stays in his position to receive.

Mark 5:36

As soon as Jesus heard the word that was spoken, He said to the ruler of the synagogue, "Do not be afraid; only believe."

To me, this shows the necessity of our part in being positioned in faith. Jesus didn't say, "It doesn't matter what you believe or whether you believe; I'll heal her anyway". He immediately corrected any temptation to deviate off that path of receiving from God. Don't get into fear- only believe, and in this case, keep believing!

Psalm 27:13

I would have lost heart unless I had believed that I would see the goodness of the Lord in the land of the living.

Choosing to believe gives us heart and prevents us giving up when discouraging words or contrary circumstances come.

It is also important that we do not pray that prayer of unbelief that ends with, 'if it be thy will'. We are meant to find out what God's will is and then pray, 'Your will be done on earth as it is in Heaven'. The prayer "if it be thy will" is a prayer for when we don't know what God's specific will for our life is. It may be like a prayer of dedication, such as 'God, if it's your will, I'll take this job' or 'go to Africa'.

James 1:6-8
But let him ask in faith, with no doubting, for he who doubts is like a wave of the sea driven and tossed by the wind. For let not that man suppose that he will receive anything from the Lord; he is a double-minded man, unstable in all His ways.

So one challenge is that in the midst of many words and much advice, that we choose to believe God's Word. Not only do we choose to believe but we choose to stay believing, even in the midst of contrary symptoms or circumstances. James indicates that to doubt is not just outright unbelief but rather, wavering between believing God's Word one moment and heeding the contrary circumstances the next. He likens it to a wave tossed backward and forwards by the winds. James warns us that to waver with doubt, means that we will not receive from the Lord- a very sobering thought!

God's Word is the truth, no matter what we experience in life. At the time when I first started teaching on healing, I was actually still suffering from the long term illness that I had experienced. I said to the Lord that I shouldn't teach on healing because I am not yet healed, and that would limit the message or cause people to question it. The Lord responded to me, "Kate, My Word is still the truth whether you are healed or not. Preach My Word".

We have to be so careful not to make the Word of God and the doctrine of healing conform to our circumstances or on whether 'so-and-so' was healed or not. If we argue from a point of someone not being healed or experiencing what God had provided for them, not saying that it is through any fault of their own, then we are, however unconsciously, making God's truth bow to the circumstances.

The Bible is absolute truth, in absolute purity, and cannot be altered in any way or for any reason. We are to, to the best of our ability, which we know is not always perfect, take the Word of God and allow it to change our circumstances, so they conform to it.

I have been in a meeting where, after presenting 'how to receive healing', someone has spoken up about how they were in faith and it didn't happen for them. They concluded that we shouldn't be telling people to believe and giving them false hope when, according to their experience, sometimes God has another way. Unbeknownst to them, in that same meeting there was another person suffering a similar condition and now doubt had come to them and they wondered if God had another path for them. If God says that He heals all and that Jesus bore sickness for all, then it's for all. If He says, that 'none shall suffer miscarriage or be barren in His land', then His will is 'none shall suffer', even if our experience is not always reflective of that.

For those who didn't receive healing on an occasion, it's important that they don't dampen the faith of others or discourage them from believing God by implying that sometimes God has a different will for them and that the healing is not for all. On the other side of this is that we need to never judge people who have not received their healing. We are not to assume that they weren't in faith but understand that some things we don't have the answers to.

PICTURE

KEEP YOU EYES ON WHAT GOD'S REPORT SAYS– KEEP ATTENDING TO WHAT HE SAYS IN HIS WORD AND NOT THE SYMPTOMS OR ANY BAD REPORT.

PAUL'S THORN

I am going to look at one other area of challenge to belief for healing before going on with our steps of faith. In teaching on healing there is usually someone in the class who will ask about Paul's thorn, and so let's get that hindrance to faith out of the way before we move on.

2 Corinthians 12: 7-10
And lest I should be exalted above measure by the abundance of the revelations, a thorn in the flesh was given to me, a messenger of Satan to buffet me, lest I be exalted above measure.

Concerning this thing I pleaded with the Lord three times that it might depart from me.

And He said to me, "My grace is sufficient for you, for My strength is made perfect in weakness". Therefore most gladly I will rather boast in my infirmities, that the power of Christ may rest upon me.

Therefore I take pleasure in infirmities, in reproaches, in needs, in persecutions, in distresses, for Christ's sake. For when I am weak, then I am strong.

In 2 Corinthians 12:2-6, Paul tells of how he was taken up to heaven, receiving an abundance of revelations from the Lord. The revelations Paul received, whether then or at other times, are revealed to us through his writing of 13 books of the New

Testament. Up till this time, the church age and all it encompasses (the new promises, power, authority and grace that we receive through Christ) was hidden. Satan came immediately to oppose him (recalling in Mark 4, that Satan comes immediately to steal the Word).

Paul states that this thorn in the flesh was a messenger of Satan. The messenger from Satan came because of the revelation, to hinder Paul from communicating the message of grace. Wherever people received the message of grace, the church changed and became empowered.

The messenger of Satan was a demonic spirit, not a sickness. Of the 176 times the Greek word 'angelos' is used in the New Testament, 147 times it refers to 'angel' or 'angels', twice 'angel's', six times 'messenger' or 'messengers' and once as 'spies'. The messenger of Satan was a demonic personality who was behind all of the trials that Paul had been experiencing, which he enumerates in the previous chapter. Wherever Paul went with the gospel, opposition rose up to hinder him. It was sent to buffet him, which basically means it sent blow after blow against him, as with winds buffeting a house in a storm.

It is good to note that his discussion of the thorn in the flesh is in context with experiencing trials and not with sickness. Paul describes in 2 Corinthians 11:22-33 how he received the 39 lashes five times, three times beaten with rods, a Roman form of punishment and even stoned to death. Stoning was only for bringing the death penalty and not for punishment alone. The victim was placed at a lower level and stones were aimed at his or her head. Paul was raised from the dead and went straight back into the city, being Lystra in Galatia, to continue his ministry. He was shipwrecked three times; a day and night in the deep; robbed; in hunger often etc. Not once in this extensive list does he mention sickness.

In Galatians 4:13, Paul does say, 'You know because of physical infirmity I preached the gospel to you at the first'. An infirmity, according to Vine's dictionary is better translated as a 'weakness, want of strength or inability to produce results' [9]. This weakness was physical but I believe that this was at the time of

Paul's first visit to Galatia, which was just after he had received the stoning at Lystra, with all those stones directed at his head.

He goes on to say in Galatians 4:15 that they would have plucked out their own eyes and given them to him. From this, some have formed the opinion that Paul had an eye disease that God refused to heal. More likely, seeing that he says nothing to that effect is that his face and notably, eyes, were still looking ugly from that stoning.

Many read 2 Corinthians 12:8-9, where Paul pleads three times for God to remove the thorn as God saying 'no'. However, God doesn't say 'no' but instead gives Paul a revelation on how to overcome, *'My strength is made perfect in weakness'*. We will discover in the next chapter that revelation always precedes the release of God's power, promises and provision.

The word strength there is the Greek word 'dunamis' which is also translated as 'power'. It's the same word for power used in Acts 1:8 when Jesus says that you shall receive power when the Holy Spirit comes upon you. It can also be translated as God's miracle working power.

The importance of the passage in 2 Corinthians 12 is the revelation that Paul gets about the overcoming grace of God. God did not remove the demon as Paul had requested but gave him His grace, or power, to overcome. So often we want to pray and have God just remove all of our problems for us, when what He wants is for us to take a hold of His power and authority and get a victory over the situation.

It is interesting to note that after this Paul writes in Ephesians and Romans about how we are more than conquerors in Christ, how we are seated with Christ above all the demonic realms, how we have the armour of God to stand against the wiles of the devil, including the shield of faith, to quench all the fiery darts of the enemy and the Word of God which is the sword of the Spirit. He got a revelation of the power and authority of God that has been delegated to us.

I believe from this Scripture, and others on redemption, that if we will take a hold of the power, Word and authority that God has given us and receive His grace, which is the power of the Holy

Spirit to overcome, then God will transform our weaknesses by His power and grace, to where we can be stronger in that area than those who are naturally strong. If you are weak in an area, you are more likely to do this and that is why Paul says that he takes pleasure in weakness, "for when I am weak then I am strong (in God)".

Jesus said to Paul, *"My grace is sufficient for you, for My strength is made perfect in weakness"*. His strength is made perfect when we are weak, because after receiving it we become strong in the strength of God and not just in mere human strength. In other words, we end up stronger than we could have ever been on our own. In Ephesians 6:10, Paul says that we are to be *'strong in the Lord and in the power of His might'*.

God's grace and mercy have always been to enable us to bear our persecutions and temptations. They are not intended for us to bear our sins and sicknesses which Jesus bore for us in our place.

BELIEVE IN YOUR HEART

B ack in 1990-1991 when I was trying to learn how to receive healing from the Lord, I was attending to the Word daily, studying it, listening to tapes on faith and healing from anointed ministers and putting into practice all that I knew to do. However, I was not getting healed.

I cried out to the Lord one day, saying, "I have done all that I know; I study your Word; I speak it out all day but I am still not healed". The Lord spoke back to me in an instant saying, "You still see yourself as a sick person." This brought me up short. What did this mean and how does it fit in with receiving the promise of healing?

This became the crucial point I found to faith, and have since found that where I was missing it, others who fail to receive healing are missing it on the same point. I often ask people who tell me that they are in faith and yet, not being healed, "how do you see your situation, your health", and the response is always, "well I see the sickness, of course".

The Bible tells us that it is what we believe with our hearts and speak with our mouths that are the essence of a faith that receives. I thought I believed with my heart because I believed the Word of God to be true, was absolutely convinced of it, could quote it and couldn't be talked out of it. Others clearly think the same thing. However, this kind of believing was clearly not enough, and wasn't positioning me, or them, to receive the promise of God. God was telling me that how I saw myself and my health was important.

Romans 10: 8-10

But what does it say? "The word is near you, in your mouth and in your heart" (that is, the word of faith which we preach): that if you confess with your mouth the Lord Jesus and <u>believe in your heart</u> that God has raised Him from the dead, you will be saved. <u>For with the heart one believes</u> unto righteousness, and with the mouth confession is made unto salvation.

So, what does it mean to believe, or more importantly, to believe in your heart, which according to Romans 10:9 is the type of belief that receives. Clearly, believing with your mind, no matter how passionately is not enough; we have to believe in the heart, which in this case is speaking of your spirit. How does your spirit believe?

Romans 10:17 says that *'faith comes by hearing and hearing by the word of God'*. The 'Word of God' here in the Greek is 'rhema', meaning the spoken or breathed word. This is where the Holy Spirit inspires or 'breathes on' the Word of God illuminating it into your spirit.

There are two revelations of the Word of God - the 'logos', which is the written Word and the 'rhema' which is this Holy Spirit inspired Word. We attend to the written Word, which contains God's will for our lives, but in order to receive His Will in specific areas, in this case healing, we need the Holy Spirit to inspire that Word to us, whereupon it becomes a 'rhema' to us. When that happens, the 'rhema' attended to and spoken out, brings the kind of faith that receives the promise.

So, we need to be in the written Word all the time in order to know God's overriding will and to be positioned for the Holy Spirit to speak to us but it is not enough to stop there. The power to bring that Word to pass in our individual lives comes as the Holy Spirit breathes on that Word we are attending to, just as He did in Creation, and then that Word releases the power to bring itself to pass. Many, like I did, are doing the right thing studying the Word of God and, yet, are still failing to receive from it and live out all that God reveals in His Word that He wants them to have because there is no power behind it.

The power comes with the 'rhema'- so then faith comes by hearing and hearing by the 'rhema' of God. 'Faith comes' which tells me that it's not always there in the first place, to receive the promise. It comes as we hear and hear the Word that the Holy Spirit has illuminated to us. To hear it, we must be speaking it out, and not just reading or studying it. Holy Spirit inspired revelation always precedes the manifestation of God's promises.

Proverbs 4:20 says to *'incline your ear to My sayings'*. Incline your ear is not just hearing the Word but also means opening the ears of your understanding by meditating on and pondering that Word. To truly hear you must listen with the ears of your spirit to what the Holy Spirit is saying to you through the written Word. In Revelation 2 and 3, when Jesus is speaking to the churches, He says, *'he who has ears to hear, let him hear what the Spirit says to the churches'*. We need to hear and not just read the Word but we also have to 'hear' with our spirits, which means, 'what is God saying to me through His Word'.

Habakkuk 2:1
I will stand my watch and set myself on the rampart, and watch to see what He will say to me, and what I will answer when I am corrected.

Habakkuk gives us an insight here on how God speaks His Word to us, remembering that the 'rhema' Word is one that is spoken or inspired to us by the Holy Spirit. He was standing his watch, spending time with God and listening to what God would reveal to him. Then, he shows the way that God does that. I will 'watch *to see what He will say* to me'.

We have to see what God is saying to us. When the Holy Spirit inspires to us that written Word that we are attending to, we start to <u>see</u> what God is saying to us and not merely believe it. I believe this is what it means to believe in your heart or your spirit. God is Spirit and He communicates to our spirit in a way that we see what He is saying. Once we see it, the power is released to bring that Word to pass.

We are to attend to the Word in such a way that we can see it, not just believe it to be true, the 'how to' of this being explained further along. We need to see God's Word and not our problem or sickness, in order for healing to manifest. For myself, as a child with a lot of health problems, I was always told how sick and weak I was, and hence, had an image of sickness in my spirit. This had to be changed by the Word of God before healing could come. No matter how real the healing power of God and redemption from sickness that Jesus has provided for us, the inner vision I had of myself was hindering me from receiving it, by keeping me off the path where His promises are received.

Now to the next verse in Proverbs 4, that gives us such insight on how faith works.

Proverbs 4:21
Do not let them depart from your eyes;
Keep them in the midst of your heart;

We are not to let the Word depart from our eyes. Now, I don't know about you but as much as I love the Bible, due to other demands on my time like family, church and work, I can't sit in front of it all day, every day, not letting it depart from my physical eyes. I think that the Holy Spirit is telling us to not let it depart from our spiritual eyes, our real vision. We need to see what God is saying to us, that is His Word, on the inside.

If I see symptoms on my body, even if they are there, more than I see what God has said to me through His Word, then the Word has departed from my eyes. It is an indicator to me that I need to attend to and meditate on the Word more in the area of God's healing promises. If I see lack rather than God's provision when a bill comes in the mail, then the Word in that area has departed from my eyes and I need to attend to the promises of God's abundant provision for those in covenant with Him.

If we don't continually attend to the Word, not just in healing, but in all areas of our lives, then the Word departs from our eyes and we start to see less than that which God has intended for us. The Lord highlighted this to me many years ago. I had spent years, daily attending to the Word of God on healing, because I needed to. After being healed for some time, I thought that I needed to stop looking at healing scriptures all the time and give more study to other areas. Even though I was reading all of the Word, most of my intense study, up to that point, had been in the area of healing.

After a couple of years, I started to develop symptoms in my body again and when I went to pray and believe in faith for healing, it did not come as quickly as I had known it to. The Word can depart from our eyes; even though we still believe it, we don't see it more clearly than what we are facing. The solution is to keep the Word before your eyes always. The Lord showed me that I would need to do this the rest of my life in order to enjoy divine health.

We keep the Word in the midst of our heart by attending to it, inclining our ears to what the Holy Spirit is saying to us, meditating on it and keeping it before our eyes. When we do that, the Word brings healing to us.

Proverbs 4:22
For they are life to those who find them,
And health to all their flesh.

The word for health here is 'marpe' in Hebrew, which means 'restoration of health, remedy, cure, medicine'. The Word in your heart is medicine, cure, and restoration of health to all your flesh.

John 6:63
It is the Spirit who gives life: the flesh profits nothing. The words that I speak to you are spirit, and they are life.

Jesus' words are spirit and life and, when they are received into our hearts, they bring His Spirit and His life into our spirits which then flows on to our mortal, physical bodies. If I could put a definition to the healing power of God, it is His life overcoming the law of sin and death.

Romans 8:11
But if the Spirit of Him who raised Jesus from the dead dwells in you, He who raised Christ from the dead will also give life to your mortal bodies through His Spirit who dwells in you.

Psalm 107: 20
He sent His word and healed them, and delivered them from their destructions.

Proverbs 4:22 tells us that the Word received into your heart *'is life to those who find them'*. That means that if we don't attend to God's Word, diligently heeding the voice of the Lord and doing what is right in His sight, seeing what the Lord is saying to us, then we fail to receive the life and healing that He has for us. Hosea 4:6 says, *"My people are destroyed for lack of knowledge"*.

Like I said before, God is waiting for us to meet Him where He is at. He can be met and His promises and power received on His path, which covers His will for us. Even when God does meet us where we are at, we find that He guides us to that place of faith in Him and positioning on His path before we receive what we desire from Him.

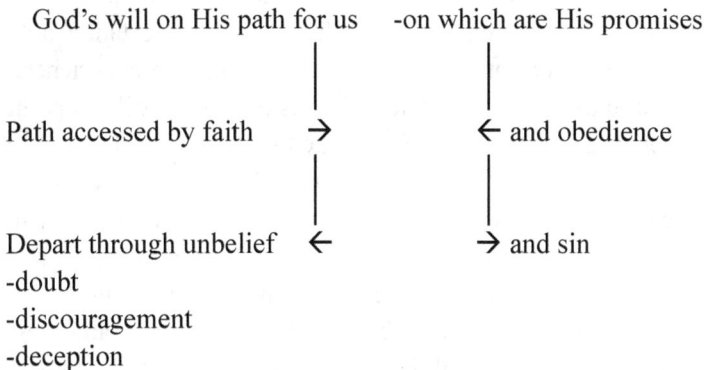

God's will on His path for us   -on which are His promises

| | |

Path accessed by faith →   ← and obedience

Depart through unbelief ←   → and sin
-doubt
-discouragement
-deception

His promises are on His path, given by grace and received through faith. We cannot position ourselves somewhere else and expect to receive from God. It sounds harsh but it does appear that God does not change His ways for us to receive from

Him that is by grace through faith, even if we are in a place of ignorance.

To me, an example of this would be Job. There is always someone who will challenge healing, saying, "Well, what about Job?" Why didn't he get healed, why did God put sickness on him or allow the devil to afflict him?

The simple answer is that God did not put sickness on him- the devil did, and God did heal him but it's just that it was preceded by bringing Job into a revelation of God as his Redeemer before that healing was released. It appeared that Job was in a place of not knowing about God's redemptive power. God didn't heal him in the place of ignorance but neither did He leave him there. He took Job on a journey into a greater revelation of God's character and when that came, the healing followed soon after.

I don't pretend to have all the answers as to why Job suffered as he did and this book is not aimed at providing a deep exegesis of the book of Job. So, the following are just a few points that I have drawn from Job that are good for us to keep in mind, before anyone starts to accuse God of being unjust or refusing to heal someone.

Job probably lived before the giving of the Law, as did Abraham. The sufferings of Job discussed in this book cover a period of only about nine months of his life. It is important to note that Job is an upright man and a wealthy man. He experienced this time of extreme trial but his life was blessed up till this point and then doubly blessed after he came through the trial.

The fact that he was an upright man shows that adversity or sickness does not mean that someone has some hidden sin in their life as Job's friends, and some Christians, wrongly imply. Sickness or adversity are present in the earth; came about because of the Fall and Satan's presence in the Earth; and most importantly find their healing or deliverance through the Person of Jesus Christ.

We don't always have the answers as to why things happen to people or why they suffer, but as we put our trust in God, we can be confident that He will bring us to a place of deliverance.

Points to consider:

1. Job lived before God's covenant and so had no written Word to bring faith, as we do. He had to operate from his own understanding and what God would reveal directly to him.

2. All His sufferings are listed under the curse of the law, which we are delivered from, in Christ. Job's suffering is a picture of what we have been delivered from. We cannot be compared to Job when we live under the New Covenant with the extraordinary blessings of what Christ has done for us.

   Job is a bit like Cornelius in Acts 10 - good, God-fearing and offering sacrifices to God, but not in a covenant position to receive all that God has for him, until Peter leads him to Christ. Job shows us that it's not enough to be good, but we need power over the devil and over sickness to avoid the likes of his suffering. We have this power now through Jesus Christ!

3. We move away from the favour and covering of God through not being in faith or obedience.

Job 3:25

"For the thing that I greatly feared has come upon me, and what I dreaded has happened to me."

Job offered up sacrifices regularly but possibly offered them in fear of judgment rather than in an attitude of faith and worship towards God. It has to be remembered that he did not have the teaching or the covenant that we now enjoy. In the Old Testament, it was faith in God that cleansed and delivered you, as you obeyed Him in offering up the sacrifice, not the sacrifice itself. Faith has always been required to receive from God.

4. The perpetrator is Satan and the deliverance comes from God (Job 1:7-12). In verses 9 and 10, Satan accuses Job of only serving God for the benefits of being blessed.

Job 1:11

But now, stretch out Your hand and touch all that he has, and he will surely curse You to Your face!"

Does God do this? No. It is the devil that strikes Job. Some say that it wasn't God that allowed it but Job by his lack of faith; that God was just observing that all that was Job's was already in Satan's hands because Job was in fear. The debate over this can be complicated. We don't have all the reasons for why people suffer, nor how much is allowed by God when our faith is tested and how much is allowed by us. In any case, under the New Covenant we are the ones who are meant to resist the devil.

5. Job believed in God and was faithful to Him but needed a greater revelation of Who God wanted to be to him. He knew God as El Shaddai, the Almighty, great and yet distant, but not necessarily as his Redeemer. He progressed in revelation throughout the book until in Job 19:25, he received the revelation 'I know that my Redeemer lives'. God is the Redeemer of all of the law of sin and death including sickness and the curse, not the author of it. It is interesting that Job received the revelation first, before he received the healing and deliverance. It's the same for us, even though the promise is there for us all the time.

God does not leave Job in his state of suffering. As he remains true to God, God leads him into a place of greater revelation of Him and restores to Job twice as much as the devil had robbed from him. By the end of Job he received revelation of what it really means for God to be Almighty – the Deliverer, Provider, All Sufficient One, the Healer. In the worst case of suffering, God was there and redeemed the situation. Nothing is too great for Him to redeem.

In Job 42:5, Job says, 'I have heard of You by the hearing of the ear, but now my eye sees you." He didn't see God with his physical eyes as his encounter with God was through the Lord speaking to him out of a whirlwind. He had a revelation of God and was seeing Him from a new perspective.

Now we will return to Proverbs 4 and 'believing in your heart'.

Proverbs 4:23

Keep your heart with all diligence,

For out of it spring the issues of life.

Proverbs 4:23 NIV
Above all else, guard your heart for it is the wellspring of life.[7]

If the Bible says, 'above all else', it must be important! Out of the heart springs the issues of life or the NIV says that *'it is a wellspring of life'*[7]. What's in your heart determines what flows out into your life. Is it healing or sickness, faith or fear, abundance or poverty, love or hate? It's not your circumstances that determine your life but what is in your heart.

We are then told, in verse 24, to guard our mouths for that is how these 'issues of life' are sown into our hearts. Jesus said in Mark 4:24, *"take heed what you hear"* in context with the parable of the sower.

<u>Two scriptural examples of this principle and a few examples of personal application of having to see what God is saying to us.</u>

The following two scriptural examples are ones that I used to apply to two of the situations that we were faced with. The first one is how to approach a situation that is impossible, or to understand that age is not a hindrance to receiving the promise of God.

1. Abraham

Romans 4:16-21
Therefore it is <u>of faith that it might be according to grace,</u> so that the <u>promise might be sure to all the seed,</u> not only to those who are of the law, but also to those who are of the faith of Abraham, who is the father of us all, (as it is written, "I have made you a father of many nations") in the presence of Him whom he believed- God who gives life to the dead and calls those things which do not exist as though they did;

Who, contrary to hope, in hope believed, so that he became the father of many nations, according to what was spoken, "So shall your descendants be".

And not being weak in faith, he did not consider his own body, already dead (since he was about a hundred years old) and the deadness of Sarah's womb.

He did not waver at the promise of God through unbelief, but was strengthened in faith, giving glory to God, and being fully convinced that what He had promised he was also able to perform.

I love how the Holy Spirit, when He inspires a teaching years later, leaves out the bits where we don't do so well. Verse 20 says that Abraham didn't waver at the promise of God through unbelief. Well, that is what he ended up doing, but the journey was not a perfect walk of faith. Therefore, it is one that we can learn from, because we don't always get it right, straight away either.

The background to this passage of faith starts in Genesis 15 and 17. God comes to Abram (as Abraham was then known), saying, "Do not be afraid, Abram. I am your shield, your exceedingly great reward." Abram's response is basically, "What good is that to me God, since that I have no child to be my heir? What is the use of blessing me so much if I have no one to pass it on to?"

God immediately promises him that one from his own body will be his heir and straight after that takes Abram outside and says, "Look now toward heaven, and count the stars if you are able to number them" and He said, "So shall your descendants be". God was telling him what to see.

The next thing that God does is to make a blood covenant with Abram as Abram asks "How shall I know that You will keep Your word to me?" Now, we don't understand a lot about blood covenants in our culture but in ancient culture, they were understood to be an unbreakable pact. When two parties entered into a covenant they were saying that they and all that they owned were at the disposal of their covenant partner should they ever need it. Attached to the covenant would be promises made that could not be broken, such was the sanctity of the covenant. The covenant was then sealed with blood and the partaking of a covenant meal. So, when God immediately initiates a blood covenant with Abram along with the promise, Abram would understand just how serious God was about keeping His Word. God was attaching His life to His promise to guarantee it.

So, Abram has a promise, God has told him what to see regarding the promise and he has a blood covenant with God. Twenty four years go by and nothing happens. In that time Abram goes a little off track, through unbelief, as in frustration Abram and Sarai try to bring the promise of God about by the work of the flesh rather than by faith which resulted in the birth of Ishmael.

Isn't it the same with us at times? We have a promise from God and a covenant sealed in the blood of His precious Son, Jesus, that guarantees the promise to us, and yet still not seeing the promise come to pass. I believe the key is seeing what God has told us to see regarding that promise.

In Genesis 17, God comes to Abram again, now 24 years later with Abram 99 years old and Sarai 89, and repeats the promise. This time both Abram and Sarah respond by laughing (Genesis 17:17 and Genesis 18:12-15). They can't see it happening!

The way that they received the promise in impossible circumstances is the same way that we receive a promise for the impossible. The NIV says of Romans 4:18, that *'against all hope, in hope he believed'*[7]. Nothing is impossible for God (Luke 1:37) and nothing is impossible to he or she who believes (Mark 9:23).

God changed Sarai and Abram's names to Sarah and Abraham. Abraham means 'the father of nations' or 'father of a multitude' which was in line with the promise God was giving Abraham. God was calling Abraham the father of many nations even before he had a child, and was teaching Abraham to do the same. It is interesting that God had made him a promise, but He still required Abraham to believe it and speak in line with the vision in order for it to come to pass. He had to call those things that did not exist (still in the future) as though they already did (past tense) in line with the way God Himself speaks.

So now I picture Abraham having to go and tell everyone that his name is now 'the father of a multitude' and that is what they have to call him from now on. He is speaking that 'rhema' over and over as he does this, faith coming by hearing and hearing by the Word of God. As he is doing this, he sees the stars in the sky and the dust on the ground (Genesis 13:16) and he recalls 'so shall your descendants be'. Now, he is starting to see what God is saying to him.

Abraham believed according to what God had already said (the 'rhema'). This is important. We are not just hyping something up or trying to manipulate God, (as if we could), to give us what we want. We speak what is already His revealed will to us, as healing is. We believe according to what He has already said.

Next, he didn't focus on the problem. He knew it was impossible. Sarah had been barren all her life and now she is ninety, and Abraham about one hundred. Abraham did not consider his own body (parallel of symptoms or weaknesses), nor the deadness of Sarah's womb (parallel of impossible circumstances around us). He did not deny the problem, but he did choose to primarily focus on the answer instead.

You need to renew your mind and see the Word in your heart to the point where you are consumed with God's truth, and not the facts of your situation. You can't focus on the problem and the answer at the same time. Only one can fill your vision, and the one that does determines what you will have. The Israelites couldn't keep their vision on the brazen serpent and their symptoms of snake bite at the same time if they wanted to be healed.

Many Christians confuse positive confession to be denial of the sickness, going around saying 'I'm not sick'. Faith is not denial but choosing to believe that God's promise is enough to override the problem that you do acknowledge exists. So, we know that there is a sickness to be dealt with; we don't deny it but choose to focus on and see the promise of God's Word instead, understanding that what we see is what we will receive.

Now Abraham, because he is speaking out that 'rhema' word over and over, choosing to focus on it (and not the contrary facts of his situation) and seeing what God has told him to see, doesn't waver at the promise of God through unbelief (Romans 4:20). He had to build up his faith to get to that point and to be 'fully convinced' that what God had promised He was also able to perform.

It was twenty four years that Abraham and Sarah had the promise and the covenant with no results, but only three months from the time that they spoke and saw in line with the 'rhema' word until Isaac was conceived. I know the timing of God comes into things as well, but I do believe that this situation highlights the need for us to believe in our hearts and see what the Lord is saying to us in order for His Word to come to pass.

Just because things don't change immediately doesn't mean that it won't happen. If you received everything from God, as soon as you asked for it, you wouldn't need faith. Faith is believing for what you cannot see with the natural eyes, and it is 'through faith and patience' that we inherit the promises of God (Hebrews 6:12). The fact that we also need patience indicates that a waiting period may be involved.

My story
At the same time that I was ill many years ago, we were also told that I would be unable to conceive children, and that I should try fertility treatment. I have a passion to see things work out in practice, previously with science and now with the Word of God. I decided that I wanted to see God do the impossible based on His Word and that here was the opportunity.

By the time God had spoken to me that, "You still see yourself as a sick person", I had already fallen pregnant three times, but all had resulted in miscarriage.

I had already sought out the scriptures that I would apply and speak into the situation, the passage in Romans 4:16-21 being one of them. Before I believe God in any area I like to get His direction from the Word. I ask the Lord what is the scripture or teaching that I need for the situation. Many years later, I will still go to my prayer closet and say to the Lord, "I will not leave until You show me Your will for the situation and give me Your 'rhema'". Once that Word comes, which it always does, I apply it to the situation, and without fail, that Word carries power and I can feel things shift from the time that Word is declared out in faith.

Now I realised that I had to move from believing and start

to see the scriptures, like Exodus 23:26, *'No one shall suffer miscarriage or be barren in your land'*, and *'against all hope, in hope he believed'*, so that he became the father (or she the mother). I started trying to see myself with a baby and, a good friend (thank you, Jane Allen), brought me a pram to help my vision.

Another thing that the Lord directed me to do was to worship in the midst of the problem. He directed me to Isaiah 54:1, where the barren woman is called to sing. I struggled with this at first; it seemed so hard to worship during such heartache, but worship releases the miraculous power of God.

Isaiah 54:1

"Sing, O barren, you who have not borne! Break forth into singing, and cry aloud, you who have not laboured with child! For more are the children of the desolate than the children of the married woman," says the Lord.

The Lord showed me that if we will worship Him in the midst of our barrenness in any area then He will turn that situation around to the place where we will be more blessed in that area (that is, more are the children of the desolate; children being a sign of blessing in the time of writing) than those who have not faced the same challenge or for whom everything had gone well in that area (characterised by the married woman).

Romans 4:20 says that Abraham was strengthened in faith, giving glory to God before he had the breakthrough. At the time, I had a card framed in my house with a Scandinavian saying on it, 'Faith is a bird that knows dawn is breaking and <u>sings while it is still dark</u>'. We have the Word to bring us faith and vision, but we also need to sing while it is still dark.

As I was praying and 'trying to see' the promise one day, the Lord gave me a vision. The background to it was that we had come from C3 church in Sydney (then Christian City Church in Brookvale) to be with a church in Canberra for a season. The vision was that I walked through the doors at Christian City Church, Brookvale, and our pastors, Phil and Chris Pringle were there, holding the hand of a little girl. The little girl was about three years old, with blond hair and blue eyes. Pastors Phil and Chris silently handed her to me, and that was the end of the vision.

The vision only lasted an instant of time and yet, it changed the whole course of that journey. As they say, a picture speaks a thousand words. I knew that as soon as we returned to Sydney and our old church, then I would have my baby. I was ready to just get straight in the car and go.

We went to our pastors in Canberra and told them that we felt to leave and go back to Sydney, but they said they felt that it was not God and that we should stay. One of those attitude and submission tests! Don't you love them? We decided to help them build the church up and go back to them again with the same request in six months. After six months, the church had grown and we were given the release to go. We literally jumped in the car, with the dog and a few boxes and left everything else behind.

Within a month of returning to Sydney, I conceived our beautiful little miracle girl, Annalise. When she was three, she looked just like the little girl in the vision with her blond hair and blue eyes. Later on, during my second pregnancy, an ultrasound was taken showing that I was completely healed from polycystic ovarian syndrome, one of the issues that had been preventing me having children, and the attached report said that I must not have had the condition in the first place because there is no sign of it now. However, the earlier report had stated a severe case of polycystic ovaries.

In that six month period in Canberra, between requests for release from our pastors, I actually had another two miscarriages. What I want to share with you now however, is the response to a situation without seeing God's promise and the response when you do see the promise.

After the first three miscarriages, I was absolutely devastated. I found it hard to pray, I was depressed and discouraged, and my emotions were like a roller-coaster. I found it really hard to step into that place of trusting God again. I was accusing God of not caring. After receiving the vision, the next two miscarriages were like a non-event. Why? It was because I already had the baby - I could see her. She was more real to me than my circumstances. Once you have that vision on the inside, and you really believe with your heart, then it is just a matter of time before it comes to pass and you know it. You already have it because you can see it!

Hebrews 11:1
Now faith is the substance of things hoped for, the evidence of things not seen.

You can feel the substance of that Word come into your spirit as you begin to see it. Once you can see it, you know you've got it and that is the substance of faith that the writer of Hebrews is talking about; the evidence that God's Word is going to come to pass in your life, before you can see it with your physical eyes.

Our circumstances rarely come into line with the vision straight away, but, once you believe in your heart, they no longer rock you because you are seeing something different and something far more real to you than the circumstance. That's the level that the Word in your heart has to get to; you see it more and it is more real to you than the contrary circumstance.

If we find that circumstances are rocking us, that we are discouraged or even complaining against God, then it is an indicator that we are not really in faith. O yes, we might believe the Word but we are not seeing it, and believing in your heart is seeing what the Lord is saying to you.

This is not to condemn or discourage us but to provide an indicator that more of the Word is needed here to bring us into that place of really believing. <u>Faith is not blind but the perception of another and far greater reality</u>. When Paul the apostle says that we walk by faith and not by sight (2 Corinthians 5:7) he is not saying that we walk blindly, not knowing or perceiving where we are going. <u>Faith sees into God's reality and walks in the light of that.</u>

It may be different for each person, the vision they hold inside, but when going to the Lord for healing, I have a vision fixed into my spirit of Jesus on the Cross. I see His suffering, the affliction laid on Him, the blood He shed for me. As I look, I think 'He is going through all of that, bearing my sickness. It's on Him and therefore, I have been set free from it." As long as I hold that vision, I am not moved by my circumstances.

Psalm 16:8
I have set the Lord always before me; because He is at my right hand I shall not be moved.

The second situation that we will look at is what to do if the situation is due to a genetic problem. I have had people come to me and say that healing is not for them because the situation they are dealing with is genetic, as if Jesus on the Cross took all our sicknesses but left the genetic ones behind.

2. Jacob
This particular story about Jacob is outlined in Genesis 30:25-43, a favourite one regarding the power of a vision. Jacob wanted leave his father-in-law Laban but Laban knew that God was blessing him through Jacob. Laban tells Jacob to name his wages and he asks for all the sheep and goats that are spotted and speckled and the brown lambs. The ones not considered speckled or spotted or the brown among the lambs would be Laban's.

However, Laban tricks Jacob and removes all these uneven coloured sheep from the flock and gives them to his sons. Now the natural law of genetics applies here. The even coloured sheep left in Jacob's care, those belonging to Laban, are going to produce even coloured progeny leaving Jacob with no wages.

God then gives a dream to Jacob showing him to take sticks of poplar, almond and chestnut, tear into the bark, making the branches appear spotty and striped. He was then to place the branches before the watering troughs, so the animals should conceive before them, when they came to drink. So Jacob put the branches up when the strong or pedigreed flocks came down to drink and breed, and removed them when the weak animals came.

Genesis 30:39

So the flocks conceived before the rods, and the flocks brought forth streaked, speckled, and spotted.

By getting Jacob to see what He was saying to him, God was able to change the genetic makeup of those animals. Now I know that this story is often used to show the power of putting a vision before the church flock, and as valid as that is, I don't believe that this is what is actually happening in Jacob's story. For literal goats and sheep are not the most spiritual of creatures and unlikely to conceive a vision from God. The vision was so that Jacob would catch the vision and thereby be able to see a genetic change take place in the flock.

In the next chapter, when he is relaying the story, Jacob reveals what God had told him to see.

Genesis 31:11, 12

Then the Angel of God spoke to me in a dream, saying, 'Jacob.' And I said, 'Here I am.' And He said, 'Lift your eyes now and see, all the rams which leap on the flocks are streaked, speckled, and gray-spotted; for I have seen all that Laban is doing to you.

Now look at what God says. He tells Jacob to see the rams are streaked, speckled and spotted, but they aren't! How often do believers say, I can't see the promise of God in my vision because I can't see it with my eyes. However, we walk by faith and not by sight (2 Corinthians 5:7). Jacob had to see what God was saying to him in order for the Word to take hold in his heart and release its power to change the situation.

My story

When Annalise, our beautiful daughter, was very young, she had a reverse bite, a condition that was genetic among the females on one side of the family, and uneven teeth. She was unable to bite any food properly as the lower part of her jaw and teeth protruded well in front of the top row of teeth, the two rows failing to connect at the front. So, she had to bite food with her back teeth which was very awkward.

We heard from other relatives of the long term orthodontic work that would be required, the wiring of the jaw and the pain, not to mention the expense. I decided that I would believe for God to do the impossible, and would take Annalise back to the dentist in 18 months time, when she would be 5 years of age. We were urged by some that we needed to act straight way with orthodontic work. One such similar case that we are aware of, resulted with astronomical orthodontic bills over many years, but with no cure.

So we prayed the scriptures over Annalise, saw her with a perfect bite and perfectly aligned teeth. When I took her to the dentist 18 months later the dentist was amazed at this child with a perfect bite and perfectly aligned teeth. She is 18 years old at the time of writing, and at every dental visit since, has been told that she has a perfect bite and will never need orthodontic work.

Now, obviously, this is not as serious as many genetic conditions that people suffer from. However, the principle is the same. If we will believe in our heart, seeing what the Lord is saying to us, and speak with our mouth, then we will be healed, understanding that healing is part of our salvation.

Now, how do we get the Word from a place of believing it, to where we can see it? It is primarily by meditating on the Word of God. Christian meditation is not like Eastern meditation. Eastern meditation is emptying your mind; Christian meditation is filling your mind and heart with the Word of God.

One of my favourite scriptures is in Joshua 1:8. Joshua is about to take the nation of Israelites into the Promised Land, with many obstacles for them to yet overcome. So, the strategy that God gives him is going to have to be extremely powerful.

Joshua 1:8
This Book of the Law shall not depart from your mouth, but you shall <u>meditate in it</u> day and night, <u>that you may observe to do</u> according to all that is written in it. For then you will make your way prosperous, and then you will have good success.

The Amplified version of the Bible reads *'that you may observe and do* '³. We are to meditate on the word until we can see it, and when we see it, we find that we automatically will do it.

We are not just to read or study the Bible but to meditate on it. The word 'meditate' (Hebrew- hagar) means 'to murmur by implying to ponder, imagine, meditate, mourn, mutter, speak, talk, utter, study'. Now God tells Joshua to meditate on the Word day and night. This might seem impossible to do along with life's demands, but I find that if you just spend some time meditating in the Word, apart from your reading and studying time, then that scripture seems to run around your head all day. I sense the Holy Spirit speaking to me about it throughout the day, thus, I am meditating on it day and night, even though I am not sitting in front of my Bible all that time.

I take a scripture to meditate on. I don't just read it but spend at least 10 minutes on the one scripture. I think about it. How does this apply to my life? What is the Holy Spirit saying to me through this scripture? I start to visualise it. How does my life look with this scripture manifested in it? I speak it out; faith coming by hearing and hearing by the Word of God. This starts to plant the seed of the word in my heart.

In the early days, Richard and I learned that meditating on the Word was the key to changing a person's life to line up with the Word of God and to position them to receive God's promises. We had so many situations that needed changing. I had fallen ill soon after we were married. In fact, the severe symptoms started on our honeymoon. We were then told about not being able to have children. We had taken out our mortgage based on my income as a pharmacist while Richard changed careers from geology to retail, which necessitated starting at the bottom of the ladder along with an associated income drop. However, now I could not work and so the finances were so tight that it looked like we would lose our house. We had a lot of opposition to us becoming Christians, bringing with it considerable challenges.

I remember going to a pastor, at a previous church, with all the things we were facing and he looked overwhelmed and just said, 'Go home and read Psalm 91'. It sounds funny, seeing that it wasn't probably the best pastoral encounter, but it was the best thing that happened to me because it forced me to push into God and His Word for myself. We need pastors and mentors, and we really need to listen to them and learn from them, but we also have to learn not to run to people every time we are in trouble, but to God. The role of a pastor or leader is not to solve all your problems but to direct you to God, Who can solve them all. People, however great they are, are never your source.

Similarly, because people seemed overwhelmed by some of the things we were dealing with at the time, and because some past issues were coming up with the infertility diagnosis, I thought that perhaps I needed counselling. Everyone else who had problems seemed to go to counsellors. I prayed about it and the Lord directed me to Isaiah 55:1-3.

Isaiah 55:2,3a
Why do you spend money for what is not bread, and your wages for what does not satisfy? Listen carefully to Me and eat what is good, and let your soul delight itself in abundance.
  Inline your ear, and come to Me. Hear, and your soul shall live.

Now, don't get me wrong, counsellors have their place when people are struggling but they are never a substitute for God and the power of His Word, described in scripture as His bread which we are to eat by hearing and attending to it.

Well, following my pastoral advice, I did go home and read Psalm 91, but also many other scriptures. It was obvious that only God could change many of the things that we were facing. I had lists of scriptures for every situation that we needed to see change in.

I would get up in the morning, feeling weak and sick, and get to the bathroom. There, on the mirror via a sticky note, was *'by whose stripes you were healed'* (1 Peter 2:24). That's right, I am healed! Immediately your focus starts to change. You don't meditate on the Word in order to get healed but to see that you already are healed. Your body or actions naturally follow the image that you have of yourself. Proverbs 23:7 states that as we think in our heart (or how we see ourselves) so we are.

Then I would get to the kitchen and there on the fridge, *'My God shall supply all your need according to His riches in glory by Christ Jesus'* (Phil 4:19). That's right! We won't lose our house or not be able to pay our bills; God will provide. Richard would drive to work, with sticky notes with scriptures written on them, all over the driving wheel. We were meditating on the Word day and night and when we started to see it God's power went to work, turning around every one of those situations, bringing us to a place of healing, provision and blessing.

Psalm 1:1-3
Blessed is the man who walks not in the counsel of the ungodly,
*   Nor stands in the path of sinners, nor sits in the seat of the scornful;*
*   But his delight is in the law of the LORD, and in His law he meditates day and night.*
*   He shall be like a tree planted by the rivers of water,*
*   That brings forth its fruit in its season, whose leaf also shall not wither;*
*   and whatever he does shall prosper.*

The leaf is symbolic of healing. In Revelation 22:2 the leaves on the tree of life are for the healing of the nations. If we will meditate on the Word of God day and night, we will be fruitful, healed and whatever we do shall prosper.

Often as I share this with people, they look at me as if to say, 'it's too simplistic; there has to be more to it than that'. The truth is God has made it within reach of all us to receive His promises and blessing by making the method easy. For all that, most people won't do it, thereby failing to experience all that Jesus purchased for them.

I love the fact that God has not made it difficult for us to receive His healing, or indeed, any of His promises. The faith of a child is enough to receive from Him. Children believe easily and receive easily. When Annalise was about twelve years old, I started having to teach her, not only was God her Healer, which she already knew, but how to receive from Him herself.

This came about one day when, after praying for healing for her, for some minor illness, she failed to receive her healing as usual. The Lord showed me that she was now ready to receive from Him herself and that He was expecting her to do the 'standing in faith'. So, I brought out the scriptures on healing and asked her to meditate on them for twenty minutes. After that, we prayed and she was healed. Since then, if the children needed healing, I would ask them to meditate on the scriptures first, thus positioning them in faith, before praying for them. I find that, in so doing, they are far more likely to be healed, and quickly.

Having your heart in the right condition

In the parable of the sower, in Mark 4, Jesus reveals four states of the heart that exist in Christendom, only one of which receives the fruit or manifestation of the promise.

Mark 4:14-20

The sower sows the word. And these are the ones by the wayside where the word is sown. When they hear, Satan comes immediately and takes away the word that was sown in their hearts. These likewise are the ones sown on stony ground who, when they hear the word, immediately receive it with gladness; and they have no root in themselves, and so endure only for a time. Afterward, when tribulation or persecution arises for the word's sake, immediately they stumble. Now these are the ones sown among thorns; they are the ones who hear the word, and the cares of this world, the deceitfulness of riches, and the desires for other things entering in choke the word, and it becomes unfruitful. But these are the ones sown on good ground, those who hear the word, accept it, and bear fruit: some thirtyfold, some sixty, and some a hundred."

The Word of God is His seed and it needs to be planted in our hearts in order for it to produce a harvest. A healing harvest requires healing scriptures, meditated on and planted in a heart free from negatives attitudes, fear, and the cares of this world, which will then produce 30, 60,100 fold what was sown.

The first heart condition is where the seed is stolen. If you just hear the word and don't give any thought or study to the message heard, then the devil comes and steals that word away.

I discovered this as a new believer. I would hear an amazing message on a Sunday and then later in the week, my brother-in-law, who was not in church at that stage, would ask what the message was on. I couldn't remember. I thought, my pastor spends his Wednesday morning seeking God for a message, receives it and after delivering it on Sunday, I forget it. If God gave him a message then surely He intended that I would receive it and put it into practice. From that time on, I have taken notes in church, even if it's a message I've heard before, so that I can go home and attend to it, thus allowing it to stay in my heart.

Mark 4:23, 24 Amplified version
If any man has ears to hear, let him be listening, and perceive and comprehend...Be careful what you are hearing. The measure (of thought and study) you give (to the truth you hear) will be the measure (of virtue and knowledge) that comes back to you, and more (besides) will be given to you who hear.[3]

Jesus said that the measure of virtue, or power, and knowledge that comes to you is directly related to the measure of thought and study that you give to the truth you hear.

The second condition of the heart is where the seed is sown on stony ground. That means that the ground has not been dug up and turned over as required to plant the seed. These people get excited over the message and believe it but their hearts are not changed by it. When a challenge comes to that word, they 'believe' for the promise and maybe even speak it out, but nothing happens. Hence, they conclude that faith or the Word doesn't work, and they stumble.

The heart has to change to accommodate the seed, just as the surface of the soil has to change and be turned over, to plant the seed. There is no seed established and no root of the Word, if the heart is not changed by that word. We have to change what we see in our hearts to line up with the Word of God.

The third heart condition is where cares, worry or thinking on the problem grow another crop at the same time that chokes the Word. It's whatever you are meditating on that plants a seed and produces a harvest. It's not enough to focus on your symptoms all day, think and speak out worry and then spend ten minutes in the Word, speaking that out. If you plant them together the thorns of worry and unbelief will grow up with your seed and choke the harvest, making it unfruitful.

Also, beware that in the absence of any positive planting weeds grow in a garden. We need to be aware of what we are meditating on, that is, thinking about, seeing over our lives and speaking. We have to remove the negative things as well as disciplining ourselves to meditate on God's Word.

The fourth heart condition is the one that produces. This is where we are disciplined to meditate on and speak the Word of God and remove the weeds of unbelief. This heart produces a great harvest from the seed that was planted, in this case, healing.

Some people feel that they need to know how God is going to bring about their healing. You don't need to understand how God will bring your harvest- you just need to do your part of planting and watering the seed.

Mark 4:26-29
And He said, "The kingdom of God is as if a man should scatter seed on the ground, and should sleep by night and rise by day, and the seed should sprout and grow, he himself does not know how. For the earth yields crops by itself: first the blade, then the head, after that the full grain in the head. But when the grain ripens, immediately he puts in the sickle, because the harvest has come."

You plant the seed of Word, and it is watered by the Holy Spirit Who breathes on that Word to make it revelation to you, and it will grow. The seed contains life in itself. The Word of God contains the life of God to bring itself to pass when believed upon.

In Romans 1:16, Paul writes '*I am not ashamed of the gospel of Christ* (the Word of God) *for it is the power of God unto salvation (*which includes healing) *for everyone who believes'*. The Word of God is the power of God when believed upon. The power to bring it to pass lies dormant, just as the life or DNA lies in a seed, until faith is applied to it. Then that seed of the Word bursts open and the life of God is released to bring that Word to pass.

Over a period of time your seed will grow (Mark 4:28) if it is cared for, first the blade, then the ear and then the fully grown plant. We need to understand that healing is often a process. Otherwise, so many get discouraged when they don't see results immediately.

Jesus reveals the importance of believing in your heart in Mark 11:22-24. The background is that Jesus, on the way from Bethany to Jerusalem, sees a fig tree and being hungry wants to eat from it. Now the tree had leaves which meant that it should have also had fruit but there is none, and so Jesus curses the tree, saying, *"let no one eat fruit from you again"*.

He goes into Jerusalem and returns again to Bethany at the end of the day, past the tree but no one has noticed any change in it. The next morning, they are passing the tree again but now they notice that the tree has 'dried up from the roots'.

Mark 11:22-24
So Jesus answered and said to them, "Have faith in God.

For assuredly, I say to you, whoever says to this mountain, 'Be removed and be cast into the sea,' and does not doubt in his heart, but believes that those things he says will be done, he will have whatever he says.

Therefore I say to you, whatever things you ask when you pray, believe that you receive them, and you will have them.

Jesus says that if we have faith, which would require that we have a 'rhema' from God, we could speak to a mountain and move it, obviously the 'rhema' Word from God having to be about moving that mountain. He is using an extreme example to illustrate a principle.

He does not say that if we just speak a word or the Word of God over and over, that we will have whatever we say. He says that firstly we have to not doubt in our heart. This means that if there is no doubt in our heart, then there is a heart that totally believes. As previously discussed, to believe in the heart is to see what God is saying to you. So, if we completely see what God is saying to us, with no doubt or contrary vision in our heart, and then we speak out of that heart condition, then we will have whatever we say.

In order for faith to operate and produce, we need a heart that sees what God is saying to us; in this context, one that sees God's complete provision for healing, coupled with a mouth speaking out that same Word.

We believe that we receive it first; that is, we see it in our heart and believe that it is done. The Word is then deposited in our spirit, and over time, we will receive its manifestation in the physical realm, as we continue to see and speak in line with it. This is not some form of mind science or thinking healing comes from the self. Rather, it's a repositioning to where we are not focussed on ourselves and our problems, but on our God and Saviour, Jesus Christ, and what He has done for us.

PICTURE

SEE YOURSELF AS A HEALED PERSON ACCORDING TO ISAIAH 53, THAT JESUS HAS BORN ALL YOUR SICKNESSES, PAINS AND WEAKNESSES AND 'BY WHOSE STRIPES YOU WERE HEALED'.

WHAT WOULD YOU BE DOING IF ALL YOUR SICKNESS HAS BEEN TAKEN AND YOU WERE HEALED- SEE IT!

SEE JESUS HAVING TAKEN THE SICKNESS OR AFFLICTION FOR YOU

SPEAK THE WORD OF GOD OUT

Proverbs 4:24
Put away from you a deceitful mouth,
  And put perverse lips far from you.

We need to be speaking out God's Word and not other words that would deceive our hearts into believing and seeing something else.

Romans 10: 8-10
But what does it say? "The word is near you, in your mouth and in your heart" (that is, the word of faith which we preach): that if you confess with your mouth the Lord Jesus and believe in your heart that God has raised Him from the dead, you will be saved. For with the heart one believes unto righteousness, and with the mouth confession is made unto salvation.

The word of God must be established in your heart and in your mouth. We believe in our hearts, and speaking the word out of our mouths is how we release the faith that is in our heart, in order for it to create.

The word 'confess' is the Greek word 'homologeo', meaning, according to Vines dictionary, 'to speak the same thing, to assent, accord, to agree with'[9]. In others words, if we are speaking out the same thing that we believe in our heart, that is, what we see on the inside, then that aspect of salvation, in this case healing, is released.

Mark 11:23

For assuredly, I say to you, whoever says to this mountain, "Be removed and be cast into the sea", and does not doubt in his heart, but believes that those things he says will be done, he will have whatever he says.

Once again the scriptures show us, this time from the mouth of Jesus Himself, that what we believe in our heart and what we speak with our mouth must agree in order for faith to work. Even if we are speaking out scriptures, if we see sickness or the problem, then healing is not released. We can see healing and Jesus' provision for us on the inside but, if we don't speak it out, the power is not released. The heart and the mouth have to work together.

2 Corinthians 4:13

And since we have the same spirit of faith, according to what is written, "I believed and therefore I spoke," we also believe and therefore speak.

The spirit of faith speaks. If we really believe something, whether good or bad, then out of the abundance of the heart the mouth speaks. In Psalm 116:10 from which Paul is quoting, the psalmist has recognised the principle in speaking the negative in a bad situation. Paul applies it in a positive manner in 2 Corinthians 4:13, that if we really believe the gospel then we will speak it no matter what persecution comes, because it is impossible to separate what we believe and what we speak. If we really believe something, then we will speak it, thus releasing what we believe into our world.

If you still see sickness or the problem, don't speak it out because that is what you will be releasing into your world. Instead, cover your mouth, get out the Word of God and start meditating on it until you see what you would like to be released into your world.

The situation may not change immediately because it takes time for your belief about it to change and line up with the Word of God but, once it does, that heart of faith and mouth combination will create the answer that you need.

Another thing that I find is important is not to be randomly or mechanically confessing out scriptures but strategically speaking them into the vision or belief of the Word that you have on the inside. You can be speaking scriptures out all day, as I was in the early days of seeking healing, and have not much happen. Remember, the heart and the mouth has to work together. So you can't have your attention in another place while your mouth is speaking out the Word and see great results. Remember, your attention needs to be on the Word; you are 'in the moment', you are seeing Jesus bearing your sickness or weakness, and then you speak the Word into that image. It's not just the heart belief or just speaking the Word - it is having the two work together!

Hebrews 11:3
By faith we understand that the worlds were framed by the Word of God, so the things which are seen were not made of things that were visible.

The things which were made were made of things not visible; that is, through the substance of faith that is the evidence of things not seen, as referred to in Hebrews 11:1. God created from a heart of faith, that faith being released by the Word, which the Holy Spirit moved on in order to form all of Creation. Then He created us in His own image.

Proverbs 18:21
Death and life are in the power of the tongue and those who love it will eat its fruit.

So when we speak from a belief in our hearts, releasing it through the words of our mouth, we release one of two things into our lives. We can speak death, the problem or sickness that we face, coupled with a heart that sees the problem or sickness, and release more of the same into our life, thus, not changing anything for the better. Or we can speak life, the Word of God, coupled with a heart of faith, and see our lives changed and the power of God's Word and promises released to us. Either way, there will be fruit, that is, results, from what we speak.

Proverbs 12:14 NIV
From the fruit of his lips a man is filled with good things as surely as the work of his hands rewards him.[7]

This is saying, like Proverbs 18:21, that we will see results from the words that we speak, in just the same way that we see results from our physical labour.

In Isaiah 57:19, God says, *"I create the fruit of the lips"*. Well, He can only create it, if it is in line will His will. However, if we are speaking His Word, then the Holy Spirit will move on it, just as He did at Creation, bringing it to pass.

Other scriptures along these lines are the following.

Jeremiah 1:12 *...for I am watching to see that My word is fulfilled.*

Isaiah 55:11 *So shall My word be that goes forth from My mouth; it shall not return to Me void, but it shall accomplish what I please, and it shall prosper in the thing for which I sent it.*

I know that it says that the Word is going forth from God's mouth, but if we will put His Word in our mouths, we will find also, that it prospers, that it produces great results in the thing for which is was sent, because God is watching over it to fulfil it.

Many years ago, I suffered a short period of depression following the birth of our second child. My heart goes out to anyone suffering this over long periods. It was like being in a black hole; I couldn't enjoy anything, even though there was nothing majorly wrong in our circumstances; I had no motivation and was always tired. I was thinking, 'what is wrong with you girl. You believed for children; God has done amazing miracles for you; you have a wonderful husband and family- what is your problem?'

Due to the lack of energy and motivation, I was not praying with the required passion and authority, and subsequently not seeing any change. Finally I got in our lounge room one night and thought, "I need to deal with this thing now with the Word of God". I was speaking out the Scriptures on healing, joy and peace and it felt like they were leaving my mouth and falling to the ground like lead. I kept speaking the Word and then was aware of this voice coming against my mind saying, "You idiot- you think that you can just speak out words and it all magically goes away."

However, I was speaking the Word of God and not my words, and His Word carries His power. After about twenty minutes, I felt this black cloud lift, rising until it moved above my head and left. I now know that it was a spiritual presence that had come against me, but the Word of God has its effect whether it is a spiritual or physical cause. A couple of times, over the next couple of months, at the end of a day when I was tired, it would try and return. Those heavy emotions and negative thought patterns would come, but as I spoke the Word out, it would quickly leave again, until it no longer returned. The Word of God accomplishes God's will and prospers in the thing for which it was sent.

James 3:6 says that the tongue defiles the whole body. We need to be careful about what we are speaking over our bodies or health. James 3:2 also says that if we were perfect in the words that we spoke, able to bridle the tongue, then we would also be able to bridle the whole body. The words we speak do affect our bodies, as well as our behaviour and direction in life.

What are you speaking over yourself? The 'joy of the Lord is my strength' or 'I'm having such a hard time'? 'By Jesus stripes I have been healed' or 'I feel so sick', 'I'm so tired'. 'I am anxious for nothing', 'the peace of God guards my heart and mind in Christ Jesus' or 'I'm afraid', 'I'm so worried', 'I don't see how this can work out'. Speak God's answer for every situation, and resist speaking out the problem or sickness.

A few examples from Scripture

Mark 5:39
When He came in, he said to them, "Why make this commotion and weep? The child is not dead but sleeping".

Jesus has come to the house of Jairus, where his daughter has just died. Jesus approaches the problem by speaking in faith and not voicing the problem. The response was that the mourners ridiculed Him. Undeterred, He puts them outside and then raises the little girl from the dead.

Too many believers are voicing their problems, calling that facing reality but, if we want the results of God then we have to do things His way. He *'calls those things which do not exist as though they did'* (Romans 4:17). He is well aware of the problem, but to overcome it He calls forth the answer that does not yet exist in the physical realm as though it already did (past tense), and in so doing, shows us to do the same.

In John 11, we see how Jesus deals with an impossible problem, that of raising Lazarus from the dead. The first thing He does is to be careful not to speak the problem, but the answer, but because the disciples aren't following what He is doing He is forced to state the problem. Later on, He will have to reinforce speaking the answer.

John 11:11-14

These things He said, and after that he said to them, "Our friend Lazarus sleeps, but I go that I may wake him up."

Then His disciples said, "Lord if he sleeps, he will get well".

However, Jesus spoke of his death, but they thought that He was speaking about taking rest in sleep.

Then Jesus said to them plainly, "Lazarus is dead".

The following verses reveal Jesus' discussion with Lazarus' sisters trying to get them to see the answer - Jesus as the resurrection and the life. Finally, after Martha advises Him that Lazarus has been dead four days (Verse 39), Jesus replies in a way, that I see is intended to shift her to believe.

John 11:40

Jesus said to her, "Did I not say to you that if you would believe you would see the glory of God".

Jesus then speaks out, thanking God that He has heard Him, stating that His statement of faith was for those listening, so that they would believe, before calling to Lazarus to 'come forth'.

Speak those things which do not yet exist in your world as though they did, based on the word of God, and the power of God will be released to bring them to pass.

Mark 11:24

Therefore I say to you, whatever things you ask when you pray, believe that you receive them, and you will have them.

The other thing about the prayer of faith, is that it is not only based on the Word of God but it is also bold, has authority and some passion in it. It's not casual or a weak and feeble prayer.

What do I mean by this? Say, you are requiring healing for influenza. You are feeling rotten, tired and weak, and your prayer is coming out in a similar way. It's got an attitude of 'I'm tired, poor me, I feel so bad'; it sounds more like a groan. Or some believers tell me that they are praying the Word and I ask them to pray so that I can hear how they are praying. They speak the Word but it's coming out in a weary, weak manner. My experience (and theirs) is, that it doesn't get a response. It has no faith in it because the prayer of faith has energy and authority behind it.

Jesus said in Matthew 11:12, *'the kingdom of heaven suffers violence and the violent take it by force'*. This is not talking about physical violence or being an aggressive believer but having a 'fight' in your prayers. The kingdom of heaven is not talking about Heaven itself but the realm of God's power and promises that He intends us to live in, made available through receiving Jesus as our Lord and Saviour. Paul says in Romans 14:17 that the kingdom of God is righteousness, peace and joy in the Holy Spirit. It also includes healing, provision, love, God's grace and mercy. God has given us the kingdom, that is, the fullness of salvation, including healing, but it is contested.

This kingdom suffers violence in that the devil or circumstances come to try and rob us of all that Jesus has made available to us through His death and resurrection, which includes health and healing. They assault the kingdom, stripping away from believers their health, provision, peace, joy, and well- being. We are not meant to sit back, passively accepting this.

The believer is on the other side of the battle, the kingdom of heaven being what is being fought for. We are to take back by force what is being stolen from us. The scripture is not talking about being aggressive with God or arrogant in our faith. We are fighting for what He has already given us, against an opposing force.

Often we ask God, "Why didn't You heal this person? Why did you allow this to happen?" The truth is that He has provided healing for the person, in His kingdom, and it has been given to every believer. He then empowers us with faith through His Word and the Holy Spirit to take hold of and maintain the kingdom. He doesn't allow it to be taken. Instead it is taken because it is contested by an opposing force.

This must never be translated into judgment on those who didn't receive healing, as them not being in faith or not having done enough. Only God could be the judge of such things. On the other hand, we can certainly never be pointing the finger of blame at God.

What we often fail to recognise is that when we received Christ and His kingdom, we entered a war, because the devil is determined to challenge us in this. As in every war, casualties occur, through no fault of their own. You don't judge casualties of war for being hit.

What we do need to do, is train people so that they have the best chance of winning. In war, those who are highly trained and understand the tactics of the enemy, have a better chance of survival. We need to be trained in the Word and not be ignorant of the devil's devices. However, even the highly trained in war can be taken despite doing the best they know. It is a war after all. It doesn't make it God's fault or mean that God is allowing it, if we miss what God says He has given us.

God is also not just sitting idly by watching believers suffer and doing battle. He came and broke the power of sickness off our lives; He destroyed the authority of the enemy over our lives; He gives us a kingdom that we could never have obtained ourselves and then empowers us to keep it. However, the fight to lay hold of what He has given us is up to us.

We are to have a fight in our spirits that says 'I am not going to be robbed in this area; I am not going to have health taken from me when Jesus has provided complete healing for me; I am not going to be in lack; my family members are not going to be lost but saved'. We take the kingdom back by force, in faith, in an attitude that refuses to lose to the devil or circumstances and most importantly, by the power of the Word of God, which is the sword of the Spirit (Ephesians 6:17).

Far too many believers I meet have misinterpreted the passage in Ephesians 6:14-18 about putting on the armour of God. Too many are going through steps, in prayer, seeing themselves putting on their armour or pretending to put on the items. That will do nothing to stop the devil. The armour of God are things that we must do, not pretend to put on. To win a battle you must be in God's truth, have the absolute assurance that you are right with Him, based solely on what Jesus has done for us and not based on our own performance, and walk in peace. Then, in verse 16, it says, 'above all, taking the shield of faith with which you will be able to quench all the fiery darts of the wicked one'. Put your shield up by boldly believing God and seeing the reality of Him and His promises to us. Believe Him!

After guarding your mind against doubt, deception and discouragement with the truth of what's been given to you in salvation, 'take the sword of the Spirit, which is the Word of God'. Speak that Word out boldly, while seeing in faith what is rightfully yours, and keep speaking and standing in faith until you get your healing back.

As a family we have shared on the times when prayer brought healing and when it didn't. Without fail, this issue has come into it. When we could feel the discomfort or a threat against the wallet, a motivation and a 'fight' came into the prayers. It's an assertion of faith against the sickness or problem. Just to clarify, it's certainly never the attitude towards our loving

God and Father. When we were casual with prayer, because the issue wasn't really bothering us too much, then healing didn't happen.

No matter how we are feeling, we need to rise up, declare the Word over our situation with authority, have some energy and passion in the prayer, and then we will find power is released.

James 5:16b
The effective, fervent prayer of a righteous man avails much.

James 5:16b Amplified version
The earnest (heartfelt, continued) prayer of a righteous man makes tremendous power available (dynamic in its working).[3]

James is relaying the story of Elijah, who, as James says, being someone just like us, prayed and the heavens shut for three and a half years, and then prayed again, and it rained. The key is the type of prayer. It is effective which means that it is a prayer of faith. It is fervent and heartfelt, which means that it has some passion in it.

By way of an example, I had a very small growth on my eyelid that was going to need to be surgically removed. As it was small and such a minor issue, I really hadn't bothered too much with it until I found out that I would need surgery. My prayers had been casual- I did believe the Word but really wasn't applying it in faith the way I knew to. As a result, I didn't experience any change. I asked my GP if he could remove it as it was starting to be a bit more noticeable and he said that it would require surgery. Now, not wanting surgery, I moved to faith. I looked at it in the mirror, saw it gone, spoke to that growth to leave, and prayed in faith with passion and authority. Then, I totally forgot about it. A month later, as I was applying mascara to my eyelashes, I suddenly realised that the growth was no longer there.

Casual, lazy or weak prayers don't work. We must pray in faith!

I'll share another example of how faith is required, by which I mean not just believing the Word but applying it with boldness, energy and authority. There is glaucoma strongly in my family line, which combined with the fact that I had suffered eye damage (now healed) at an early age, put me in the high risk category. After forty, all family members are meant to be tested for the disease.

I had my eyes tested and the pressures in them were high (an indicator for glaucoma) and so they asked me to come back in two weeks to get them retested. I didn't think too much about it, assuming that it would be okay and so really didn't put any focussed prayer into it. The tests, two weeks later, showed extremely high pressures and I was advised to see an ophthalmologist immediately. I said, "Give me another two weeks, and redo the test", knowing that now I needed faith filled prayer and not casual prayer. On that note, we never need casual prayer because it doesn't work and therefore is nothing more than some religious exercise. The optometrist argued that I needed to see a specialist straight away, but I told them "another two weeks".

In that two weeks, I focussed on the Word, prayed in faith, by which, once again, I mean not just any old prayer but Word filled, energy filled, authority filled prayer. When my eyes were tested again two weeks later, the pressures were back to normal and have remained that way at subsequent annual check-ups.

My husband, Richard, was healed from Raynaud's phenomena, an incurable condition where the circulation to the extremities is so restricted that it causes pain, blueness or sometimes whiteness, and numbness upon exposure to the cold. It had resulted in him not being able to swim, not being able to go in the surf which was something he loved and not being able to be out in the cold. It was painful to teach at Bible College because of the air conditioning. It was also meant to restrict him from doing the water baptisms at church because of the cold water, although he did them anyway.

As winter approached, the symptoms were getting worse. Richard really got the fight in his spirit that was necessary for healing to take place. He refused to allow things to remain the way they had been diagnosed. Being winter, it would have been too easy for him to remain inside with the heating for his morning prayer time. Instead, he rugged up and went out into the cold, refusing to not be able to do it, declaring the Word of God over and over. Overall, it had been six months, but healing came pretty soon after he got that real fight that said, 'I am not going to have this anymore'.

PICTURE

THE MOUNTAIN OF SICKNESS BEING REMOVED FROM YOUR BODY ACCORDING TO THE WORDS OF YOUR MOUTH- SEE THE EXPECTED FRUIT OF THE WORDS YOU SPEAK

ACT ON THE WORD

Proverbs 4:25-27

Let your eyes look straight ahead, And your eyelids look right before you.

Ponder the path of your feet, And let all your ways be established.

Do not turn to the right or the left; Remove your foot from evil.

Now, we need to walk out the healing process. As we consistently attend to the Word of God, meditating on it until we see it and speaking it out, it will direct our actions to line up with that Word. Sometimes, healing takes a lot longer than you would like, to manifest. The fact is that although God has given us the fullness of salvation, it is not always walked out quickly. For example, we are delivered from sin but do we overcome it in the physical realm in a day? No, we have to 'work out our salvation with fear and trembling' (Philippians 2:12). We have to allow what God has already given us to be worked out in our lives through faith, which more often than not is a process.

James 2:17

Thus also faith by itself, if it does not have works is dead.

James 2:17 Amplified version

So also faith if it does not have works (deeds and actions of obedience to back it up) by itself is destitute of power (inoperative, dead).[3]

It helps to think of works in this context as actions or behaviour that accompanies faith. If you really believe something then it will change you, in accordance with the change in your heart, leading you to act on it. Faith without actions is incomplete. More often than not our actions, circumstances or health just naturally change in response to a heart of faith linked with a mouth speaking out the Word of God. The blessing comes with the action; all the other steps are to get us to a place where we can obey.

Joshua 1:8

This Book of the Law shall not depart from your mouth, but you shall meditate in it day and night, that you may observe <u>to do according to all that is written in it.</u> For then you will make your way prosperous, and then you will have good success.

Often the Lord will direct you to do something that either you could not do before or an act of obedience that may seem silly but your faith and action of obedience, together, release the healing that you are believing for. Often, I believe, He is shifting you out of a mindset, where you saw yourself as not being able to do what you now can do.

Years ago, after hearing God say to me, "you still see yourself as a sick person', I started to really meditate on the Word, seeing myself healed and asking the Holy Spirit to show me what He was saying to me through the scriptures. One day, soon after, I felt Him ask, "If you were healed, what would you be doing right now". I looked outside at a messy garden that had been neglected since we had moved in after our marriage. I thought, 'I would be gardening' (not a thought I get very often).

I felt the incentive to go outside and start gardening. Now, up to this point, I had only been able to do very simple activity and after ten minutes of it, I would need an hour or two's rest. The muscles throughout my body had been extremely weak.

I went outside and started gardening. Then I started to move rocks, as the garden had an extensive rockery, that I didn't want. The next thing I knew, it was three hours later and Richard had come home from work, saying "what are you doing?" I had worked for three hours in mid-summer heat, weeding and moving rocks, without any need for a rest. From that day, healing came into the muscles of my body and I was able to start exercising and working again, without regular rests. It began the first stage of healing from an illness that had affected every organ of my body, and it steadily continued from there.

The first time our daughter, Annalise, stood in faith, by herself, was as a young girl, when she badly tore some ligaments in her leg and, after scans, was told that she would be on crutches for about six weeks. Two days later, we were going away on an annual weekend get-together with friends from church, where the favourite activity for the kids was to go tubing or water skiing behind a friend's speed boat.

From the Thursday evening when she had the accident, Annalise was praying healing scriptures and seeing herself running without the crutches. On the Saturday morning, she decided to go on the tube anyway as it didn't require use of her leg, and when she got off it, decided to act on her faith and not use the crutches any more. It hurt faintly, but as she kept walking on it, the pain left and her ankle was healed. The crutches had only been needed for two days.

This area of acting on your faith often needs prayerful consideration as it has resulted in many believers taking foolish steps. Often believers hear that they need to act on their faith and then, throw away medication that they need or their glasses, only to find that the healing has not been released or occurs over a period of time, and now they are in trouble. This is often because they have not taken the time to get the Word in their hearts first, until they can see it, and so no power is released to bring about their healing.

Don't feel like you have to discontinue medication without medical advice or throw away glasses. Your healing, as it manifests, will be evident in medical tests as well as in your physical well-being and treatment can be adjusted according. This is especially important if the healing occurs over a period of time.

Another issue is the pressure, from others telling you, that you need to discontinue medical treatment in order to have faith or be healed. I don't believe the Lord is hindered by whether medical treatment is being used or not while waiting for divine healing to manifest. What I have seen is many who are on medical treatment, even including chemotherapy, be healed while many who shun it, in the name of faith, not be healed.

Our role is not to impose our judgments on others, saying for example, "You shouldn't be taking medication". Our role is to get them on God's path of grace; that is, help them to believe. Referring back to that path, if we push people to do something that they are not comfortable with, they can move into fear or be subject to doubt, which moves them out of faith and, hence, out of position to receive from God. Speak the truth to them, don't impose your conditions on them and encourage them to overcome doubt, deception and discouragement. Help people to be positioned to receive from God. It's the position of faith and not whether they take medication or not that leads them to their healing.

I find that to really be sure of what to do and when, a believer must stay close to the Holy Spirit in prayer and you will find that He will direct your steps, and when He directs them, the power will be there and you will not stumble. Many times where people received healing from Jesus, they were responding to His specific directions for them, rather than the general Word alone, and then, as they acted, healing was released.

Luke 17:14 The healing of the ten lepers
So when He saw them, He said to them, "Go, show yourselves to the priests." And so it was that as they went, they were cleansed.

One returns to thank Jesus, and Jesus said to him "Arise, go your way; your faith has made you well." The Amplified version says *'your faith (your trust and confidence that spring from your belief in God) has restored you to health.'*[3] Jesus attributes the healing he received to his faith that responded in action to Jesus' specific directions.

John 9:6, 7
When He had said these things, He spat on the ground and made clay with the saliva; and He anointed the eyes of the blind man

with the clay. And He said to him, "Go, wash in the pool of Siloam" (which is translated, Sent). So he went and washed, and came back seeing.

It took a step of faith for a blind man with mud on his face to find his way to the pool and wash. Once again, he was acting on a specific direction given to him by Jesus that, as he responded, released his healing.

Mark 3:1 and 5

And He entered the synagogue again, and a man was there who had a withered hand....

And when He had looked around at them with anger, being grieved by the hardness of their hearts, He said to the man, "Stretch out your hand." And he stretched it out, and his hand was restored as whole as the other.

It took faith for the man to act in an atmosphere of hostility from the religious leaders and to not argue that he couldn't do it. He didn't just act how he thought he should act but in response to Jesus' specific instructions, and was healed.

There are healings where the person has acted, not in response to the Lord or the leading of the Holy Spirit, but out of a strong inner conviction. However, because they are acting in response to a changed perception of their condition, I would surmise that they are still acting out of a heart of 'seeing' faith.

Mark 5:25-34

Now a certain woman had a flow of blood for twelve years, and had suffered many things from many physicians. She had spent all that she had and was no better, but rather grew worse. When she heard about Jesus, she came behind Him in the crowd and touched His garment. For she said, "If only I may touch His clothes, I shall be made well."

Immediately the fountain of her blood was dried up, and she felt in her body that she was healed of the affliction. And Jesus, immediately knowing in Himself that power had gone out of

Him, turned around in the crowd and said, "Who touched My clothes?"

But His disciples said to Him, "You see the multitude thronging You, and You say, 'Who touched Me?'"

And He looked around to see her who had done this thing. But the woman, fearing and trembling, knowing what had happened to her, came and fell down before Him and told Him the whole truth. And He said to her, "Daughter, your faith has made you well. Go in peace, and be healed of your affliction."

Now I don't know all the particulars of the situation but it says that this woman heard about Jesus. Now, perhaps she had heard that others had touched the hem of his garments and been healed, for she said *"If only I touch His clothes, I shall be made well"*. That is a very specific thought and so I imagine that she could see herself touching his garments as others had done and receiving her healing. So, she believed and most likely could see it, considering the specifics of how she believed her healing would come. She had spoken it, but now, had to act. She acted because she believed, but if she hadn't acted on what she believed, then nothing would have happened. Now, as an unclean woman, she was not allowed in crowds. She would have had to push her way through the crowd with everyone knowing that she was unclean and not allowed there. She acted like a healed woman.

Her faith drew healing power from Jesus as it positioned her to receive what He was there to give. Jesus felt her touch of faith, different to the touch of all the others around Him and said *"Who touched My clothes?"* Note, He didn't say, "Who touched Me" but specifically identifies the person as the one who touched His clothes. Probably, only one person was there to consciously touch His clothes, rather than to touch Himself. She would know that He was speaking of her.

Many people want to touch Jesus but it is the touch of faith, the touch that is specific in what it wants to receive from Him, that does receive. Jesus actually didn't initiate this healing, the woman did. She positioned herself in a place of faith that drew the healing power that was flowing from Jesus. Jesus said to her,

"Your faith has made you well".

The healing of the blind man, Bartimaeus, is recorded in Mark 10:46-52. He hears that Jesus is passing by and cries out to Him, and crying all the more for His mercy as others told him to be quiet. Jesus commands for him to be called and then Bartimaeus does this amazing thing.

Mark 10:50

And throwing aside his garment, he rose and came to Jesus.

What's so amazing about that? In that day, those who needed to beg for a living, such as this blind man, had a specific garment that identified them as such. By throwing aside his garment, that previously Bartimaeus needed in order to make a living, he was showing that he was convinced that he would be healed. He got up, acting like one who was healed; like one who had no need of that garment.

After asking him what he wanted Jesus to do for him, Jesus tells him, "Go your way, your faith has made you well" (Mark 10:52). Jesus didn't even have to pray for him or lay hands on him. Bartimaeus' faith positioned him to receive the healing that God had for him, in the Person of Jesus.

In Jesus, the 'power of the Lord was present to heal them' (Luke 5:17). In the finished work of Jesus on the Cross, the Word of God and the person of the Holy Spirit, the presence of the Lord is always there to heal us. Faith positions us to receive it.

Years ago, after sharing on healing at an interfaith fellowship meeting, I concluded with a general prayer as I had been told not to lay hands on people. Afterwards, two ladies came up to me. One had been healed of a broken ankle and the other had had a swollen arm from a spider bite, and the redness, swelling and pain had disappeared. The presence of the Lord was there to heal them and their faith, through the hearing of the Word, positioned them to receive their healing. They didn't even need someone to lay hands on them.

In conclusion of this section, we need to attend to the Word of God until we believe it in our hearts or we see what the Lord is saying to us. That is the key issue to receiving healing. If we get that right, everything else just follows. Out of the abundance of the heart the mouth speaks, and then, the heart and mouth combined cause an automatic shift in our body or how we act.

PICTURE

SEE YOURSELF DOING WHAT YOU COULDN'T DO BEFORE- WHAT WOULD YOU BE DOING IF YOU WERE HEALED- SEE IT

6

RECEIVING HEALING THROUGH COMMUNION

....

Our New Testament Communion meal has its roots in the Passover meal of the Old Testament. The Old Testament speaks prophetically about Jesus – a lot of what we understand about Jesus and our salvation is through the types and prophecies of the Old Testament. A type, among other things, is a prophetic symbol, as of an Old Testament event prophesying about an event in the New Testament (e.g. the blood of animals used to cover sin in the Old Testament is a type of the blood of Christ, in the New Testament, which removes sin from us).

God instituted the Passover when He was bringing the Israelite people out of Egypt. Everything that He specified for them to do in the Passover, in Exodus 12 was symbolic of what Christ would do on Calvary.

Moses was a type of Christ, our great Deliverer. Under God's instructions, Moses has requested of Pharoah to let God's people go – nine times he had refused and each time Egypt suffered a plague. Exodus 12:12 tells us that each of the plagues, ten in all, were specifically directed against one of the Egyptian gods. Finally God had sent Moses to warn Pharoah that if he again refused to allow the Israelites to leave Egypt, there would be a plague that would take the life of the firstborn of every household, as well as the firstborn of all of their animals. This being a judgment for sin, meant that God now had to provide protection for His own people so that the judgment would 'pass over' them.

God's people were instructed to take a male lamb 'without blemish', kill it and take its blood and 'strike' it or apply it to the two side posts and upper door post of their houses. They were then to remain inside the house (a type of the protection we have in being committed to the house of God) and eat the flesh of the lamb, roasted with fire, and unleavened bread and bitter herbs.

In the covenant meal, the body or the flesh of the lamb provided healing for the people because Psalm 105:37 tells us that *'there was not one feeble person among their tribes'* as they were brought out of Egypt. That is, 600,000 men plus women and children, perhaps two million people, coming out of harsh slavery and labour, and deprivation, with not one sick or weak among them. They were full of the lamb that represented the Lamb of God and they were healed. They also came out of Egypt as one covenant people.

Everything specified in the Passover in Exodus 12 is symbolic of what Christ would do on Calvary.

1 Corinthians 5:7
Christ our Passover is sacrificed for us

John 1:29 (John the Baptist speaking of Jesus)
Behold! The Lamb of God who takes away the sin of the world.

1 Peter 1:19
(we have been redeemed).. *with the precious blood of Christ, as of a lamb without blemish and without spot.*

The symbols in Exodus 12
1) The Lamb itself, its flesh and its blood symbolise Jesus Christ, His body and His blood.

1 Corinthians 5:7
Christ our Passover is sacrificed for us.

2) The lamb specifically had to be roasted with fire (verse 8, 9). Fire is symbolic of judgment, and so, judgment was coming

upon the lamb in their place. Similarly, the judgment due to us came upon Jesus, as our Substitute. In referring to Jesus, Isaiah 53:8 says, *'He was taken from prison and from judgment.'*

3) None of the lambs bones were to be broken (Exodus 12:46) and Jesus' bones were not broken, as was customary for crucifixion victims (to speed up death by increasing pressure on the upper body and respiration), because He was already dead under the weight of our sins and sicknesses.

4) The bread had to be unleavened. Leaven or yeast symbolises sin and bread represents Jesus (the bread that was broken at the Last Supper represents Jesus; in John 6:35, Jesus said *"I am the bread of life")*. Therefore, unleavened bread represents Jesus' sinless life. He was without sin and yet He took our judgment.

5) The bitter herbs were symbolic of the bitterness of slavery and, in subsequent Passovers, were to remind the people of the fact that God had delivered them. In Communion, we are reminded that we were delivered from the bitterness of the law of sin and death.

In Matthew 26:26-28 and Luke 22:20, Jesus Himself explains to His disciples that He is the Passover Lamb, as they celebrate the Passover meal together. The Passover feasts were different to the initial Passover. They reclined in seats (as opposed to sandals on feet, staff in hand and eating in haste ready for flight), feasted, sang psalms and celebrated what God had already done. It wasn't a fight that they were about to have but a celebration. Our Communion is like that, a celebration feast that God has already saved and delivered us. It is not a work of the flesh that we do in order to try and get forgiven, healed, or delivered. It has already been done and we receive it through faith.

Communion

1 Corinthians 11:23-30

For I received from the Lord that which I also delivered to you: that the Lord Jesus on the same night in which He was betrayed took bread; and when He had given thanks, He broke it and said,

"Take eat; this is My body which is broken for you; do this in remembrance of Me." In the same manner He also took the cup after supper, saying, "this cup is the new covenant in My blood. This do, as often as you drink it, in remembrance of Me." For as often as you eat this bread and drink this cup, you proclaim the Lord's death till he comes.

Therefore whoever eats this bread or drinks this cup of the Lord in an unworthy manner will be guilty of the body and blood of the Lord. But let a man examine himself, and so let him eat of the bread and drink of the cup. For he who eats or drinks in an unworthy manner eats and drinks judgment to himself, not discerning the Lord's body.

For this reason many are weak and sick among you, and many sleep.

1 Corinthians 11:29, 30 Amplified version
For anyone who eats and drinks without discriminating and recognising with due appreciation that it is Christ's body, eats and drinks a sentence (a verdict of judgment) upon himself. That (careless and unworthy participation) is the reason many of you are weak and sickly, and quite enough of you have fallen into the sleep of death.[3]

Just like the Old Testament people of God received healing when they ate the body or the flesh of the lamb, so too are we to receive healing, by faith, when we eat the symbol of the body of Jesus, our Lamb, represented by the bread in Communion. If you take Communion without understanding it, or as outlined in the passage, you are not in an attitude of faith or love, then you don't receive the benefits that it provides. God's promises are there for you and you don't earn them by taking Communion properly, but they are received by faith. Therefore if you are in need of forgiveness or healing, and you are not in faith, you don't receive the forgiveness and healing that you require and, hence, remain in a place of judgment or sickness. It is not a case of God judging you for not taking Communion properly but, you are not receiving its benefits through taking it in the proper attitude.

	God's blessings on the path	
	• given by grace forgiveness • healing • release from judgment	
You position yourself on the path by both faith and obedience	·····························▶	Beyond the path forgiveness and healing aren't accessed, leaving you in judgment or sickness

In this passage, I sense Paul's frustration. It's like he is saying, "If you really understood the power of what Jesus did, that is available in the Communion meal when it is taken properly, then you wouldn't be sick and certainly wouldn't die prematurely". He says to those not discerning the Lord's body and understanding what God has made available to us, 'for this reason' many are sick and weak or have died, despite healing being there for them.

I can identify three sacraments that God has instituted for the church and I find that when God institutes something, it has a divine purpose and divine power attached to it to bring that purpose to pass.

In water baptism, God's purpose is that we will leave behind the old life and be raised up out of the water, as Christ came up out of the earth, empowered by the Holy Spirit to live in 'newness of life'. When done in faith, that is exactly what happens and people find the power to leave behind the things of the past, sin, and afflictions. The decision to follow Christ and leave behind the old way of life, is made on the altar call, but the divine power to live out that decision comes at water baptism.

With the baptism in the Holy Spirit, God's purpose is that you will receive power to be His witnesses (Acts 1:8) and for all believers to receive power for ministry and, when done in faith, His power comes to do just that.

In Communion, God's purpose is that you will receive the benefits of the Cross, notably forgiveness, healing and deliverance, and when taken in faith, His power comes to do just that. I believe that there is a greater power released when we do it with the elements, than just standing in faith alone for a breakthrough.

There are two key attitudes, those of faith and love, in the taking of Communion.

Faith

Partaking of the bread in Communion.

In 1 Corinthians 11:24, when Jesus took the bread and broke it, He said *"Take, eat; this is My body which is broken for you; do this in remembrance of Me."*

Jesus' body was 'broken' with sin, sickness and disease, and every time that we take the bread in Communion we are to remember, or meditate on the fact that 'surely He bore our sicknesses and carried our pains' (Isaiah 53:4), and receive by faith the healing that He has provided for us.

Therefore, recalling the steps of faith we have already discussed, in Communion we are to:

1) Bring to remembrance, attend to and believe the Word of God (1 Corinthians 11:24)

2) Believe in your heart

See Jesus having borne your sickness on your behalf and see yourself healed.

3) Speak it out to release our faith

1 Corinthians 11:26 states that we are to '*proclaim the Lord's death until He comes*'. We are to speak out the benefits provided for us through the death and resurrection of Jesus.

The bread and the wine, or grape juice, may only be symbols of the body and blood of Jesus, but the Israelites received healing by partaking of such symbols. Some believe that as we take the elements of the bread and wine (or grape juice) that they literally become the flesh and blood of Christ. This is not so, nor does it need to be. As you identify the symbols with Christ, acknowledging that He was our Substitute, God sees it as done and responds as if it were actually Jesus' body and blood, and we receive their benefits just the same.

4) Act on your faith before you see the physical manifestation of the promise.
Don't create some action to prove that you have faith – that's a work of the flesh if you make it happen. The best way to think of it is, "If I really believe that I have been healed, how does that belief affect how I act?" It will create an attitude of thanksgiving and praise.

Many Christians believe that Communion is solely for us to remember that Jesus died for our sins but, if that were the case, there would be no need for us to take the bread. The Bible is very clear that only the shedding of blood can atone for or, in Jesus' case, remove sin. This is represented by the wine or juice and, so, if sin were the only issue in Communion, we would only need to take the wine or juice and not the bread.

Leviticus 17:11
For the life of the flesh is in the blood; and I have given it to you upon the altar to make an atonement for your souls; it is the blood that makes an atonement for the soul.

Matthew 26:28 (Jesus speaking)
For this is My blood of the new covenant, which is shed for many for the remission of sins.

Hebrews 9:22
And according to the law almost all things are purified with blood, and without shedding of blood there is no remission.

The bread represents Jesus' body, broken for us in bearing sickness, weakness and pain, thus making healing available to us. Remember, that as we stand in faith, using the elements in the

Communion meal, there is a far greater release of God's power for healing, than just by standing in faith alone.

Love

God is not interested in us just going through the motions or doing religious rituals but in connecting with Him and His power, out of which we are to live as He did towards others. Reading 1 Corinthians 11 in context, we see that the members of the Corinthian church were not walking in love toward one another. There were divisions (verse 18), and cliques, and the wealthy members were feasting on the bread and getting drunk on the wine at Communion (or their 'love feast') while the poorer members were going without (verse 21). God is love and we are hindered in receiving from Him if we do not walk in love towards our fellow mankind. Galatians 5:6 states that faith works <u>by love</u>.

Paul instructed us that we fail to receive through Communion when we don't discern the Lord's body. Discerning the Lord's body is not only understanding what the bread and wine represent and applying faith to them, but, also, understanding the church as one body. It was Jesus' body that bore our sickness and pains, but it is also His body that is His church. Jesus bore sickness once for all, but there should not be sickness on His body now. Therefore, there should ideally not only be no sickness in members of the body of Christ but, also not in the collective body, the Church. If we are one body, then there is absolute necessity for unity amongst members of the Body of Christ.

1 Corinthians 10:17

For we, though many, are one bread and one body; for we all partake of that one bread.

So, to eat and drink 'in an unworthy manner' in this context is to not be giving thought to our relationships with others.

Matthew 5:23-24 (Jesus speaking)

So if you are offering your gift at the altar, and there remember that your brother has something against you, leave your gift there before the altar and go; first be reconciled to your brother, and then come and offer your gift.

We need to be taking care of our relationships, as much as is possible with us, and dealing with any wrong attitudes before we come to worship God or partaking of the Communion meal. We are to understand that we are not just entering into a covenant with God, but also one with His Body, the Church. We are one covenant people, just as the Israelites, through the Passover meal, identified themselves as one covenant people.

Some people are concerned that they are hindered by relationships that are not going well but which they have no control over. The person may be too difficult to fellowship with, for a variety of reasons, particularly those people who are abusive. Or, the other party may not be open to reconciliation. You can only do your own part. Walk in love and forgive others, and live at peace with others <u>as much as is possible with you</u>, and your fellowship with the Lord will not be hindered.

Partaking of the wine or grape juice in Communion
In 1 Corinthians 11:25, Jesus says that the cup is the new covenant in His blood. When two parties entered into a covenant they were saying that, they and all that they owned were at the disposal of their covenant partner, should they ever need it. In the covenant, promises were made, that were absolutely binding. The covenant was sealed with the partaking of a meal, the exchange of food to symbolise 'I am in you and you are in me' and was sealed with blood, in some form or another, to symbolise the exchange of life between them.

In Jesus, God made a new covenant with mankind in which He declared, 'all that I am and all that I have is available to you should you ever need it'. Note that the covenant is a two way thing, and in entering into it, our response back to God needs to be exactly the same. We don't just receive Him as Saviour but as Lord, choosing to give our lives, abilities and obedience back to Him, out of gratitude for all that He has done for us. Attached to the new covenant are all the promises of God that are 'yes and amen' in Christ (2 Corinthians 1:20).

At the foundation of that covenant with God, is our need for forgiveness and the removal of the sin that separates us from God. We can't come into covenant or communion with Him while we are still separated from Him. The wine or grape juice represents the blood of Jesus that has provided not only forgiveness of sin, but our salvation and deliverance from the kingdom of darkness into the kingdom of God.

Colossians 1:13, 14
He has delivered us from the power of darkness and conveyed us into the kingdom of the Son of His love, in whom we have redemption through His blood, the forgiveness of sins.

Revelation 13:8 tells us that Jesus is the Lamb slain from the foundation of the world. Before God created man, He knew that man would sin and so, He had a plan to redeem man even before He created him. When Adam sinned, the human race as a whole fell from glory and was subjected to the law of sin and death and to the influence of Satan who had the power of death (Hebrews 2:14). After Adam fell, God's first response was to put blood between man's sin and judgment. God Himself shed the first blood in a type of Christ when He clothed Adam and Eve with the skins of animals. The skins would have been dripping with blood, which covered their sin and stood between them and judgment.

This set a precedent for the animal sacrifices of the Old Testament, beginning in Genesis 3:21, which covered man's sin because they represented the blood of the Messiah to come. The people's faith in the blood sacrifice kept them from judgment and the power of the devil as our faith in Christ's blood protects us.

However, when Jesus came and shed His divine blood, man's sin was not only covered but removed. Jesus blood effectively removed all sin because it represented His bearing of sin on our behalf, once for all, and by association, the bearing of the law of sin and death and all of the judgment due to us.

Jesus' blood in removing sin and delivering us from the law of sin and death, also removed the authority of the devil and his power, for believers who exercise faith in what Christ has done for them.

There is power, protection from Satan and deliverance from Satan in the blood of Jesus. Satan has no power where there is no sin. As His time on earth was drawing near the end, Jesus said, *"for the ruler of this world is coming and he has nothing in Me"* (John 14:30). The devil couldn't touch Him because He had no sin.

We are forgiven of sin and declared righteous, through faith in Christ's sacrifice and choosing to walk after the Spirit and not after the flesh or sinful desires. When you do sin, it is essential to repent quickly and pray the power of the blood of Christ over yourself, to get back to that place where Satan has no entry point into your life.

Often, it's not just sin, but life, circumstances and stress can open up doors for the enemy. If we are anxious, fearful, angry or in unforgiveness, the devil can enter, bringing affliction, even though Jesus has paid the price for us to be free. God doesn't just leave us without the answer. He has provided the power of Jesus' blood to not only forgive the sin but also break the power of the devil over our lives.

Hebrews 2:14, 15 New American Standard version
...that through death He (Jesus) might render powerless him who had the power of death, that is, the devil; and might deliver those who through fear of death were subject to slavery all their lives.[10]

John 12:31 (Jesus speaking)
Now is the judgment of this world; now the ruler of this world will be cast out. (by the blood of Christ about to be shed)

Romans 8:2
For the law of the Spirit of life in Christ Jesus has made me free from the law of sin and death. (the law of sin and death had been used by Satan to keep man in bondage to sin and it's effects).

So, how does this have an application for healing in the taking of Communion? There are times when an illness or disability is due to a demonic spirit or a spirit of infirmity, these being dealt with by the blood of Jesus rather than His bearing of sickness in His body. There are many times in Jesus' ministry where instead of laying hands on the person, He instead cast a spirit out of them. This, however, does not mean that every occasion where those conditions occur, that it is due to a spirit; just that it can occur.

Spirits of infirmity are not only seen in sickness or disability but also in cases of depression (once again, not in all), oppression, mental illness, calamities, adverse circumstances and all the curse of the law upon mankind.

Luke 13:16

So ought not this woman, being a daughter of Abraham, whom Satan has bound – think of it – for eighteen years, be loosed from this bond on the Sabbath.

Jesus was healing a woman bowed over for 18 years who had a 'spirit of infirmity' (verse 11), that is, she was bound by an evil spirit.

Acts 10:38

How God anointed Jesus of Nazareth with the Holy Ghost and with power, who went about doing good, and <u>healing all who were oppressed of the devil,</u> for God was with Him.

1 John 3:8

For this purpose the Son of God was manifested, that He might destroy the works of the devil

The works of the devil are sin and all of its consequences including sickness.

With respect to the works of the devil upon mankind, Revelation 12:12 says *'For the devil has come down to you, having great wrath, because he knows that he has a short time.'* However, the previous verse shows the weapon that we have against all the works of the devil.

Revelation 12:11

And they overcame him <u>by the blood of the Lamb</u> and by the word of their testimony.

Satan and all of his works are overcome through the blood of Christ and by our faith in what Christ has done for us. The testimony we give is not referring to our life testimony, as powerful as that is, but to us bearing witness with our heart and mouth to what Christ has done. This is how we apply the blood of Christ to our lives, by faith.

As with every other benefit of the Cross, God's protection and deliverance does not happen automatically. Jesus' blood cleansed all sin for all of mankind forever, but it is only when we apply faith to what His blood has done that we receive the benefits. In Exodus 12:23 with the Passover, when the people applied the blood of the lamb, that represented the blood of Christ, to the doorposts of their houses, God would not allow the destroyer to come into their houses to destroy them.

Each day, I apply the blood of Christ, by faith, to our lives and every aspect of our world, fully trusting its power to protect us from all the power of the devil. I remind the devil that he has no right to come into our house and put sickness or any affliction upon us, and I speak out the relevant scriptures, remembering that the power is released through speaking the Word of God.

This is why we take the wine in Communion, so that we can bring to remembrance what Jesus' blood has done in setting us free, not only from sin, but also from all the power of the devil and the law of sin and death. In this way, there is healing available through the wine as well as the bread, which we receive, along with all the other benefits of Christ's death, through faith. So, Communion is a prime opportunity for us to receive, by faith, all the benefits of Christ's death for us, in particular forgiveness, healing and release from any demonic bondage.

Keys in taking Communion
1. In 1 Corinthians 11: 28, Paul says, *"let a man examine himself"*. Under the old covenant, the Israelites had to remove all leaven, which was symbolic of sin, from their houses before partaking of the Passover meal (Exodus 12:19). In the same way, we are to look into our hearts for sin and repent of it. We are to

understand that we are communing with God, identifying that He is in us and we are in Him.

2. We are to walk in love because faith works by love. Forgive anyone who has sinned against you. Under the terms of a blood covenant, what you receive from your covenant partner, you must be prepared to give when it's needed. We receive forgiveness from God and give it back to His Body when needed. Whatever we receive from God, mercy, forgiveness, healing, grace, we are to give out to the body of Christ, His church.

3. Recall all that Jesus has one for you and 'proclaim His death' by confessing, that is, speaking out the benefits of His death for you and receiving them by faith. So, Communion is a prime opportunity to receive forgiveness of sin, healing, deliverance, strength and wholeness.

The Lord's Supper must never become simply a ritual, but it is a divinely appointed encounter by which you may appropriate today all that Jesus has provided through the work of the Cross. Just as the Israelites had to apply the blood and eat the flesh of the lamb for themselves, we have to apply the blood and body of Christ to our lives in order to receive the benefits. We do this through faith.

I want to share with you a story from Helen, a very dear friend, regarding her revelation of the power that is received through Communion. Like so many, it is not a story of an instant healing but a journey with a faithful God, Who leads us into the healing that He longs for us to enjoy but also doing other works of character development along the way.

Helen was inspired by the Holy Spirit, through hearing the teaching of Kenneth Copeland, to start taking Communion each day. She didn't know why the Lord wanted her to do this but she obeyed. Helen had been born with a hole in the heart, which had been fixed, and then received a pacemaker at 21 years of age. After becoming a Christian and then going to Bible College, she had experienced a great healing following the healing course there and the receiving of prayer, and her heart was found to be beating on its own.

Every fifteen years, a pacemaker is replaced and the doctor decided to replace it anyway, and the pacemaker was turned up.

So, now she had the pacemaker combined with her normal heart rate, which triggered Atrial Fibrillation, for which she had to take Warfarin and other medication. Her pastoral advice was to stand on the Word of God but also do what the doctors advised and to surround herself with a few faith-filled people to stand for her healing. Wisely, she didn't tell everyone.

Normally, it would be expected that she would have very low energy levels but Helen believed, through the taking of Communion, that 'those who wait upon the Lord shall renew their strength' (Isaiah 40:31). She was not sick for one day, had no side effects from the Warfarin, which is unusual and, after prayer by my husband Richard, her blood pressure went from raised to normal. She also experienced healing for emotional issues during that time.

A few years later, Helen had two operations for the Atrial Fibrillation, which were unsuccessful. Despite this, she felt from the Holy Spirit to give a gift to the surgeon. There were young doctors around at the time and she saw the looks on their faces that seemed to say, 'poor woman; she didn't get healed'. When she walked out from the surgeon's room, she felt the Holy Spirit say to her, "walk".

Helen has been walking ever since, often four kilometres a day. She goes up and down a cliff in the bush near her home as she goes on her prayer walk. She leads an incredibly busy and fruitful life, always entertaining and reaching out to others. Helen is one of the most energetic people that I know and she is really well.

Helen still takes Communion daily. She says that she uses it to focus on the Cross and thank God for the works of the Cross. She says that it has brought humility and a better understanding of Jesus' sacrifice. It has brought her into a closer relationship with Him. God has strengthened her, brought deliverance and covenant promise, thankfulness, healing, forgiveness, protection, energy, vitality, a sound mind and freedom. The great journey all started with Communion.

PICTURE

AS YOU TAKE COMMUNION, SEE JESUS, WHO HAS TAKEN ALL OF YOUR SIN AND ALL OF YOUR SICKNESSES AND PAINS.

SEE YOURSELF FREE FROM THEM.

SEE THAT THE DESTROYER MUST PASS OVER YOU BECAUSE OF THE BLOOD APPLIED TO YOUR HOUSEHOLD.

7

MINISTERING HEALING

....

W e need to understand that Jesus has intended for <u>every</u> <u>believer</u> to be involved in the area of ministering to the sick, not just those who have a healing ministry. We are all called to share our faith with others and yet, not all will be evangelists leading thousands or more to Christ. The fact of not being an evangelist, and not seeing large numbers saved in one meeting, does not mean that we can sit back and not reach out to those who don't yet know Christ, with the gospel. We are still called to preach the gospel.

Paul says in 1 Corinthians 14:39 to *'desire earnestly to prophesy'*, implying all have the potential to, through the baptism of the Holy Spirit. This does not make one a prophet, who has a special grace from God in this area, and can foretell future events in the church and the earth at large. Not being a prophet, however, doesn't mean that you can't prophesy.

In the same way, there are those who have gifts of healings and miracles who have a special grace to minister powerfully in the area of healing, seeing greater numbers of healings than most believers. This does not mean that those who don't have such ministries, can't be involved in healing the sick. In fact, it is essential that the Body of Christ at large be mobilised in this area that is so dear to the heart of God. In the same way that Jesus used healings to bring people to hear the gospel, our reaching out to others with the healing grace of God will open hearts to hear the gospel.

I am going to go through with you what I teach the students in our Bible College, on how you can bring God's healing power to another, and get yourself positioned in God to be used by Him in this way. I have no greater joy than to see the excitement in students as they get the realisation that they can do this, and see healings in others and often, their loved ones, and know that God wants to use them.

I repeat that you do not need to have a ministry, be in leadership or hold any particular position in your church for you to be used in the area of healing. The work of the minister, pastor, teacher and other ministries is to equip every believer, for them to do the work of the ministry (Ephesians 4:11, 12). The ministers are just the teachers and trainers for the Body of Christ so that they can be equipped to do the work.

Ephesians 4:11-12

And He Himself gave some to be apostles, some prophets, some evangelists, and some pastors and teachers, for the equipping of the saints for the work of the ministry, for the edifying of the body of Christ...

It goes on to say in Ephesians 4:16 that as every part does its share, it causes the growth of the body. I am so grateful to my pastor, Dr Phil Pringle, for years of teaching this truth to our congregation and that so many, including ourselves, have been released into doing the works of God.

I don't intend to cover every aspect of healing here but to provide a basic guide for every believer to be able to step into the area of healing the sick. We need to understand that we have a commission from God Himself to do this. We have been given His authority to do it. So now we need to learn how to receive the power to do it and the means of transferring that power.

THE COMMISSION TO HEAL THE SICK

Matthew 28:18-20

And Jesus came and spoke to them, saying, "All authority has been given to Me in heaven and on earth. Go therefore and make disciples of all the nations, baptizing them in the name of the Father and of the Son and of the Holy Spirit, teaching them to observe all things that I have commanded you; and lo, I am with you always, even to the end of the age." Amen.

This is known as the Great Commission, Jesus' final words to His disciples. They were to go into all the world and make more disciples, just like themselves, teaching those believers, as Jesus had done for them.

John 8:31, 32

Then Jesus said to those Jews who believed Him, "If you abide in My word, you are My disciples indeed. And you shall know the truth, and the truth shall make you free".

Firstly, Jesus says that the marker of a disciple is that they abide in His Word. That means they don't just visit it occasionally or use it to press flowers in. If you abide somewhere, then it is your principle place of residence. You are there, in residence, a lot of the time. Sitting in church or having an irregular devotional time, in both prayer and the Bible, does not make one a disciple.

A disciple has chosen a lifestyle of separation to God, devoting themselves to the Word and prayer, just as the disciples did in the book of Acts. This is important to understand because the following promises are to disciples and not just to those who have a more casual Christian walk. If you have a more casual devotional life, this is the time to change that. Jesus called for you to be a disciple, not just to 'be saved'.

What is also important to note is that being a disciple is not based on your position in the church, that is, what title you have, and whether you are a leader or not. It is a relationship with Jesus available to every single believer, irrespective of your position or call in life.

If you are a disciple, then Jesus said that you will know the truth. The word for truth here, according to Strong's concordance is 'to perceive, understand, recognise, gain knowledge, realise, come to know or the recognition of truth by personal experience'[2]. Biblical knowing of truth is to see it and experience it. It is never enough just to have cerebral knowledge alone. Jesus said that when we know His truth in our experience, then it will set us free.

Now, Jesus didn't intend to have only twelve disciples doing His will in the earth for a short period in history but many disciples operating throughout the earth until He returns. Too many have believed that healing was only with the original twelve disciples and therefore, throughout the church age so many have not been healed because Christians were thinking that they couldn't do it.

Nothing could be further from the truth. Jesus needs His whole church mobilised in this area in order to reach the sick and dying in this world, whom He cares for so much. He went to extraordinary lengths to provide healing for them but He needs His church to be releasing it in the earth today, in order for the sick to be healed.

John 17:18

As You sent Me into the world, I also have sent them into the world.

If you look at Jesus' ministry, He preached the gospel of the kingdom, taught the people how to relate to God and others, healed the sick, raised the dead and cast out demons. He sent out His disciples to do what He did, which from the gospels and the book of Acts, we can see they did.

Matthew 10:1

And when He had called His twelve disciples to Him, He gave them power over unclean spirits, to cast them out, and to heal all kinds of sickness and all kinds of disease.

Matthew 10:7, 8

And as you go, preach, saying, 'The kingdom of heaven is at hand.' Heal the sick, cleanse the lepers, raise the dead, cast out demons. Freely you have received, freely give.

Mark 3:14

Then He appointed twelve, that they might be with Him and that He might send them out to preach, and to have power to heal sicknesses and to cast out demons.

Now, Jesus is in Heaven, the original disciples are in Heaven, and He is in need of disciples here and now who can be sent to do what He did.

John 14:12

"Most assuredly, I say to you, he who believes in Me, the works that I do he will do also; and greater works than these he will do, because I go to My Father.

Too many argue today that we can't operate in that same healing power that Jesus and His disciples did. Well, Jesus Himself is saying that you can. He said that if we would believe, remembering that He is not talking about head knowledge but a belief that sees and knows by experience, then we will do what He did. How amazing is that!

If we are careful to operate according to His ways, then we can be used by God to do His works in the earth today. Jesus healed the sick and so, you can heal the sick. Jesus cast out demons and so you can cast out demons. Jesus raised the dead and so you can raise the dead. Notice He said to His disciples, 'Heal the sick, cleanse the lepers, raise the dead, cast out demons'. He didn't say to pray to God to do it for you; He said for His disciples to do it.

Jesus also said in Matthew 10:8, *"freely you have received freely give"*. We must never minister healing for personal gain or personal glory. We minister out of gratitude for all that Jesus has done for us, entirely to His glory, and for the joy of seeing someone receive their healing.

The greater works Jesus mentioned relate to the greater number, as long as the church will obey Him in this area, and also to the fact that our ministry includes the greatest miracle of all, that being, bringing a person into salvation and being 'born again'. This had not yet been made available at the time of Jesus' speaking, He having not yet gone to the Cross to secure that salvation for us.

According to Matthew 28:18, all authority has been given to Jesus, and in that authority He says "Go", to His disciples. The authority and power that have been delegated to us will only work as we are in total submission to Christ, the Head of the Body, and doing ministry according to His ways. Now, Jesus, our Head, has His Commission recorded also in Mark 16:1-18.

Mark 16:15-18
And He said to them, "Go into all the world and preach the gospel to every creature. He who believes and is baptized will be saved; but he who does not believe will be condemned. And <u>these signs will follow those who believe</u>: In My name they will cast out demons; they will speak with new tongues; they will take up serpents; and if they drink anything deadly, it will by no means hurt them; <u>they will lay hands on the sick, and they will recover</u>."

Jesus Himself is telling us that if we will believe Him that we will lay hands on the sick and they will recover. This happens as we operate in the authority that comes through His name, by the same power He Himself operated in, the power of the Holy Spirit, and through the laying on of hands.

PICTURE

YOU MINISTER TO THE SICK, IN THE SAME WAY JESUS DID, AND IN HIS NAME; WHEN YOU LAY HANDS ON THE SICK THEY RECOVER

AUTHORITY TO HEAL IN
THE NAME OF JESUS

We have been commissioned by God to heal the sick. It is His will. However, when executing the will of another, on their behalf and in their absence, we need an authority, right or a power of attorney (in the human sense) to do so.

Jesus has given us the right to use His name to establish what has already been given to us by God. Jesus has already provided fully for the forgiveness and healing of every person. He has provided for all authority over the powers of darkness. He has secured all the promises of God for us in the New Covenant sealed in His blood.

He has then also given us the 'power of attorney' to execute these things on His behalf, originally verbally, but now in written form in the Bible. If you were to look at the meaning of 'power of attorney', as it relates in the legal world, it means to act as a representative on behalf of another to look after their personal or financial affairs. Jesus has given us the right to act as His representative on the earth, doing His will, healing the sick and casting out demons, just as He did. This authority is exercised through the right that we have been given to use the name of Jesus.

Authority is the right to do something rather than the power to do it. Policemen who direct the traffic during rush hour just raise their hands and the cars stop. These people do not have the physical power to stop those vehicles if the drivers chose not to stop. They don't use their own strength to stop the traffic; they have authority that is invested in them by the government they serve. People recognise that authority and stop their cars. We have been given the authority to tell sickness or the devil to go and they must leave because we are backed up by Jesus, Who gave us that authority.

We don't have the power to destroy sickness. Jesus has already done that for us. We have the authority to tell sickness to go, in Jesus' name. We are not responsible to heal the sick; we are responsible to exercise the authority given to us.

I discovered how this authority works one day when seeking the Lord for healing. I had torn the intercostal muscles between my ribs, which was very painful. It coincided with a time when I was struggling with some teaching that I was hearing about commanding the will of God to be done. I was questioning it, having obviously misinterpreted what was being said, and was thinking, 'We can't command God; this can't be right'.

I was praying for God to heal me and distinctly felt a 'no' in my spirit. I thought, 'This can't be right; I know that God heals all the time; the answer is never 'no''. The Lord directed me to a passage in Isaiah 45:11. Now, before you correct me on it not being in context, I know it's not. This scripture has nothing to do with this teaching but for all that, it's the one the Lord directed me to and it's the one that He used to speak to me.

Isaiah 45:11 says, *'And concerning the work of My hands, you command Me'*. The Lord said, "Command your healing to be done". I argued, "Lord, I can't command you". However, He showed me that we are not commanding Him but rather, we are to use the name of Jesus to command the things that God has already given us, by grace, to manifest in our world and not just ask Him to do it for us. We are not commanding God, but the release of what is already His will, what He said He has already given us, such as healing.

I commanded healing into those muscles in the name of Jesus, and an instantaneous healing took place. I learnt something that day. So often, we are asking and praying for God to do things, when, as far as He is concerned, He has already done them. If we are praying for something that He has already done, we are to command it to be released in the name of Jesus. If it is something He has not already done, then we pray and ask the Father, also in the name of Jesus. We're never commanding God.

Philippians 2:9-11
Therefore God also has highly exalted Him and given Him the name which is above every name, that at the name of Jesus every knee should bow, of those in heaven, and of those on earth, and of those under the earth, and that every tongue should confess that Jesus Christ is Lord, to the glory of God the Father.

Jesus has the name above every other name, and when His name is spoken in faith, by a person operating in faith, then sickness and demons have to bow to His name. Note that the power is specifically in the name of 'Jesus'. Often Christians are praying something more vague, like, 'in Your name'. We need to use the name of the One who has authorised us- His name is Jesus. The power is released in His name, Jesus, and not by some allusion to it.

Mark 16: 15-18
And He said to them, "Go into all the world and preach the gospel to every creature. He who believes and is baptized will be saved; but he who does not believe will be condemned. And these signs will follow those who believe: In My name they will cast out demons; they will speak with new tongues; they will take up serpents; and if they drink anything deadly, it will by no means hurt them; they will lay hands on the sick, and they will recover."

In Jesus' name, believers will cast out demons and heal the sick. We are called to do the works of Jesus for Him, in His absence, already having His approval and authority in His name.

John 14:13, 14 Amplified version
And I will do [I Myself will grant] whatever you ask in My Name [as presenting all that I Am], so that the Father may be glorified and extolled in (through) the Son.

[Yes] I will grant [I Myself will do for you] whatever you shall ask in My Name [as presenting all that I Am].[3]

John 14:11-14 The Message Bible

Believe me: I am in my Father and my Father is in me. If you can't believe that, believe what you see—these works. The person who trusts me will not only do what I'm doing but even greater things, because I, on my way to the Father, am giving you the same work to do that I've been doing. You can count on it. From now on, whatever you request along the lines of who I am and what I am doing, I'll do it. That's how the Father will be seen for who he is in the Son. I mean it. Whatever you request in this way, I'll do. [8]

This is not talking about when we pray to the Father in the name of Jesus, as in John 15:16 and John 16:23, and the Father answering our prayer. In this passage Jesus is talking about praying in His name, and He, not the Father, doing it. This is our prayer of releasing God's will to be done on earth as it is in heaven. We pray the release of His will, in the name of Jesus and Jesus says He will do it.

Note, in the above passage in the Message Bible, that it works when we are praying along the lines of who Jesus is and what He is doing. It is to release His will not ours. The Amplified version of verse 14 brings out that to ask in Jesus' name is to present all that He is. Well, if we present all that He is to sickness, then sickness has to leave and healing will take place. If we present all that He is to a demon, then that demon must flee.

An example of this is found in Acts 3:1-10

Acts 3:1-10

Now Peter and John went up together to the temple at the hour of prayer, the ninth hour. And a certain man lame from his mother's womb was carried, whom they laid daily at the gate of the temple which is called Beautiful, to ask alms from those who entered the temple; who, seeing Peter and John about to go into the temple, asked for alms. And fixing his eyes on him, with John, Peter said, "Look at us." So he gave them his attention, expecting to receive something from them. Then Peter said, "Silver and gold I do not have, but what I do have I give you: In the name of Jesus Christ of Nazareth, rise up and walk." And he took him by the right hand and lifted him up, and immediately his feet and ankle bones received strength. So he, leaping up, stood and walked and entered the temple with them—walking, leaping, and praising God. And all the people saw him walking and praising God. Then they knew that it was he who sat begging alms at the Beautiful Gate of the temple; and they were filled with wonder and amazement at what had happened to him.

Peter responds to the man with, "what I do have I give to you". He had the name of Jesus to give and that was all that was needed. He was about to speak healing in the name of Jesus, presenting all that Jesus is to that man's disability, which brought about his healing. Note that Peter did not ask God to do the healing for him, but commanded its release in Jesus' name.

Healing prayer offered in Jesus' name brings the presentation of all that Jesus is. In addition, Jesus had said that when such prayer was given, Jesus Himself would do it. The result was the same miraculous healing, as if Jesus Himself had done the healing. Isn't that what He said would happen?

John 14:12
"Most assuredly, I say to you, he who believes in Me, the works that I do he will do also; and greater works than these he will do, because I go to My Father.

Obviously, Jesus works would not be done by any human ability but by the presentation of all that He is, through His name, with Jesus doing the healing through the presence and power of the Holy Spirit.

Jesus also said that we would cast out demons in His name (Mark 16:17, Mark 10:7).

Luke:10-17-20

Then the seventy returned with joy, saying, "<u>Lord, even the</u> <u>demons are subject to us in Your name.</u>"

And He said to them, "I saw Satan fall like lightning from heaven. Behold, <u>I give you the authority</u> to trample on serpents and scorpions, and <u>over all the power of the enemy,</u> and nothing shall by any means hurt you. Nevertheless do not rejoice in this, that the spirits are subject to you, but rather rejoice because your names are written in heaven."

The disciples are excited at the operation of authority in Jesus' name. The results are the same as if Jesus Himself had ministered. Jesus warns them not to get into a place of pride because of this. Let's face it, it's not because of how great we are that people are set free or healed, but because of how great Jesus is and what He has done for us. It is an honour to serve Him and people, and to be used to do His will, and we need to stay operating in an attitude of humility.

James 4:7 says that we are to submit to God, resist the devil and he will flee. The authority over powers of darkness works from the foundation of a life submitted to God. If a person is not operating in God's will or is involved in sin, the authority made available to believers will not have its effect. There is a story in Acts 19:13-16 that dramatically reveals that the demonic spirits know who has the right to use Jesus' name, that is, those who are born again and in faith, and those who do not.

Acts 19:13-16

Then some of the itinerant Jewish exorcists took it upon themselves to call the name of the Lord Jesus over those who had evil spirits, saying, "We exorcise you by the Jesus whom Paul preaches." Also there were seven sons of Sceva, a Jewish chief priest, who did so.

And the evil spirit answered and said, "Jesus I know, and Paul I know; but who are you?" Then the man in whom the evil spirit was leaped on them, overpowered them, and prevailed against them, so that they fled out of that house naked and wounded.

It is an honour given to believers to have the right to use the name of Jesus. Jesus' name is not something that we casually add on to our prayers without giving it thought, nor neglect it altogether, praying merely, "in Your name". We are called to pray in His name, presenting all that Jesus is, against sickness and demons, and releasing healing and deliverance, and Jesus has declared that He will do it.

PICTURE

SEE THE PEOPLE YOU ARE PRAYING FOR BEING HEALED AND SET FREE

IN EXACTLY THE SAME WAY AS IF JESUS HAD PRAYED FOR THEM

BECAUSE, THROUGH YOU,

JESUS IS BEING PRESENTED AND

JESUS WILL DO IT.

THE ANOINTING
THE POWER TO HEAL

To do the works that Jesus did, we are going to need the same power that Jesus operated with. When Jesus was on earth He did not minister as God but as a man anointed by God.

Philippians 2:6, 7 NLT
Though he was God, he did not think of equality with God as something to cling to. Instead, he gave up his divine privileges; he took the humble position of a slave and was born as a human being.[11]

The NIV version puts it:

Who, being in very nature God, did not consider equality with God something to be used to his own advantage; rather, he made himself nothing by taking the very nature of a servant, being made in human likeness.[7]

Jesus, though being God, the second member of the Trinity, gave up His divine privileges to come to earth for a season. The NIV brings out that He came to us in the very nature of God and yet without the advantages of God. He came without the power of God. Up until the time of Jesus' baptism, when the Holy Spirit came upon Him like a dove, Jesus did no miracles, no mighty works of God. In fact, in John 14:10, speaking of His ministry that followed that time, Jesus said, *"The Father who dwells in me does the works"*.

Matthew 3:16

When He had been baptized, Jesus came up immediately from the water; and behold, the heavens were opened to Him, and He saw the Spirit of God descending like a dove and alighting upon Him.

However, from the time that the Holy Spirit came upon him, He did so many miracles and healings that the apostle John says in John 21:25 if they were all written that the world could not contain the books that would be written.

Luke 4:1

Then Jesus, being filled with the Holy Spirit, returned from the Jordan and was led by the Spirit into the wilderness,

Luke 4:14

Then Jesus returned in the power of the Spirit to Galilee, and news of Him went out through all the surrounding region.

After the Holy Spirit came on Jesus He was filled with the Holy Spirit. Immediately afterward, the Spirit lead Him out into the wilderness to face what verse 13 describes as every temptation by the devil. Having overcome every temptation that He faced He returned in the power of the Spirit.

Having the power of the Spirit is the anointing to do the works of God. Being filled with the Spirit is essential but not necessarily enough to operate in the power of the Spirit. The power of the Spirit can only come on a life that is separated unto God, a person who has overcome in the area of sin. He is the Holy Spirit and cannot come on an unholy life.

Jesus then declares that the anointing of God is having the Spirit of the Lord upon Him. He then reveals what that anointing will do.

Luke 4:18, 19

"The Spirit of the Lord is upon Me, because He has anointed Me
To preach the gospel to the poor; He has sent Me to heal the brokenhearted,
To proclaim liberty to the captives and recovery of sight to the blind,

To set at liberty those who are oppressed; to proclaim the acceptable year of the Lord."

Acts 10:38
"how God anointed Jesus of Nazareth with the Holy Spirit and with power, who went about doing good and healing all who were oppressed by the devil, for God was with Him".

Matthew 4:23, 24
And Jesus went about all Galilee, teaching in their synagogues, preaching the gospel of the kingdom, and healing all kinds of sickness and all kinds of disease among the people.

Then His fame went throughout all Syria; and they brought to him all sick people who were afflicted with various diseases and torments, and those who were demon-possessed, epileptics, and paralytics; and He healed them.

He healed them all by the power of the Holy Spirit now upon Him. If Jesus operated as man anointed by the Holy Spirit, then will we not only need to be filled with the Spirit but also have the power of the Spirit to do the works that He did, remembering that this is what Jesus said we would do (John 14:12)?

Now when the apostles received the baptism of the Holy Spirit they too received the power to do the works of God.

Acts 1:8
But you shall receive power when the Holy Spirit has come upon you; and you shall be witnesses to Me in Jerusalem, and in all Judea and Samaria, and to the end of the earth."

The word power is the Greek word 'dunamis' which can also be translated as 'God's miracle working power, great might or great strength'. Many think from this verse that we receive God's power to do 'witnessing', that is, to speak about Christ. That is only part of it. The scripture says that we receive His power to be His witness. We become the witness.

We find out what Jesus' witness was when John the Baptist, from prison, asks if He is the one that they were waiting for. If we are to be a witness to Jesus then we must be a witness to what He would do. Therefore we must do the works that He did by the same Holy Spirit who was upon Him.

Matthew 11:4, 5
Jesus answered and said to them, "Go and tell John the things which you hear and see: The blind see and the lame walk; the lepers are cleansed and the deaf hear; the dead are raised up and the poor have the gospel preached to them.

This is evidenced in the lives of the disciples and not just the original twelve. The Holy Spirit on them produced the same witness as the Holy Spirit upon Jesus.

Acts 5:15, 16
so that they brought the sick out into the streets and laid them on beds and couches, that at least the shadow of Peter passing by might fall on some of them. Also a multitude gathered from the surrounding cities to Jerusalem, bringing sick people and those who were tormented by unclean spirits, and they were all healed.

Acts 19:11, 12
Now God worked unusual miracles by the hands of Paul, so that even handkerchiefs or aprons were brought from his body to the sick, and the diseases left them and the evil spirits went out of them.

One of the definitions of the word 'anointing', according to Strong's Concordance, is 'to be rubbed in'[2]. The anointing becomes rubbed into a person or an inanimate thing like a cloth or even Peter's shadow. On contact with that person or thing the stored anointing is transferred to the one needing healing.

Both Peter, in Acts 9:36-42, and Paul, in Acts 20:9-11, raised people from the dead. This healing ministry was not just for the apostles but also the works of Jesus are seen through Stephen and Philip who were deacons in the early church.

Acts 6:8

And Stephen, full of faith and power, did great wonders and signs among the people.

Acts 8:5 -8

Then Philip went down to the city of Samaria and preached Christ to them. And the multitudes with one accord heeded the things spoken by Philip, hearing and seeing the miracles which he did. For unclean spirits, crying with a loud voice, came out of many who were possessed; and many who were paralyzed and lame were healed. And there was great joy in that city.

Like these disciples, if we are to do the works that Jesus wants us to do then we will need to not just to be filled with the Spirit, but have the power of the Spirit upon us. We can't do the works of God in our own ability.

Ephesians 1:17-20

..that the God of our Lord Jesus Christ, the Father of glory, may give to you the spirit of wisdom and revelation in the knowledge of Him, the eyes of your understanding being enlightened; that you may know what is the hope of His calling, what are the riches of the glory of His inheritance in the saints, and <u>what is the exceeding greatness of His power toward us who believe,</u> according to the working of His mighty power which He worked in Christ when He raised Him from the dead and seated Him at His right hand in the heavenly places,..

Paul is praying for the church in this passage in Ephesians and included in that prayer is the desire that we would have a spiritual revelation of, that is according to verse 18 that we will see it, the incredible power that has been made available to us who believe. Paul calls it the 'exceeding greatness of His power'. Well, we know that is how the power of God is when He works it but, Paul is saying here that it's the power directed towards those who believe. He then describes the measure of that power available to us. It is the same measure of power that God exerted when He raised Jesus from the dead, when He had just borne all the sins, sicknesses, pains and weaknesses of all mankind and death itself. That is more than enough power to deal with any sickness we are confronted with. We receive this exceeding greatness of His power through receiving the same Holy Spirit Who came upon Jesus.

Luke 24:49

Behold, I send the Promise of My Father upon you; but tarry in the city of Jerusalem until you are endued with power from on high."

John 14:16, 17

And I will pray the Father, and He will give you another Helper, that He may abide with you forever—the Spirit of truth, whom the world cannot receive, because it neither sees Him nor knows Him; but you know Him, for He dwells with you and will be in you.

The Greek word for another, 'allos', means 'one besides, another of the same kind'. Jesus was saying 'I will send One besides Me but this other will be the same kind as Me'. The Holy Spirit does what Jesus would do if He were physically present. Jesus said in John 16:7 that it was better for us if He went away, because then He would send the Holy Spirit to us, Who could be with each one of us all the time, unlike Jesus, Who wouldn't have been able to if He remained down here on Earth.

The Holy Spirit is not just the power of God. He is the third member of the Trinity, with all the characteristics of a divine personality. In fact, He is just like Jesus. So someone just like Jesus comes to dwell on the inside of you when you are filled with the Spirit, and someone just like Jesus empowers you when you receive the anointing. The anointing is really the Holy Spirit, who is God on the earth bringing Himself upon your life, and with His presence comes His power and ability.

The Holy Spirit comes on a life that is set apart to God. I am about to outline some important keys to you but it is important to note that they are part of a whole lifestyle that is consecrated to God. When the Holy Spirit came on Jesus and later the disciples, He came on a life that was dedicated to God. This is a person who is pursuing holiness, overcoming in the area of sin and temptation, walking in love, walking in obedience and being faithful with what God has asked us to do at any stage in our walk with Him. We will also need to host the presence of God through prayer and meditating on the word.

1. Pursue holiness and overcome sin

1 John 1:6
If we say that we have fellowship with him, and walk in darkness, we lie and do not practice the truth.

1 John 2:6
He who says he abides in Him ought himself also to walk just as He walked.

Firstly, we need to be someone who is pursuing holiness which also does not come through our own strength and works but through receiving God's grace or power through the Holy Spirit. However, we are the ones who have to make the choices to separate ourselves from things in this life that we know are not right before God. We will need to be careful what we are watching, what we are listening to and what we practice in thought, attitude and action. As we saw with Jesus, the power of God came upon Him when He faced temptation and overcame it. We will have to overcome in the area of sin, to be holy to have God's anointing on our life. For more about overcoming sin, read the chapter on 'The hindrance of sin, especially unforgiveness'.

If Jesus were sitting in your lounge room with you or in front of your computer would you watch what you are watching? If Jesus were in the room would you speak the way that you do? Well, God the Holy Spirit is right there with you, although, if we choose to grieve Him with our choices His manifest presence is quenched or removed.

2. Walk in love

We will need to make choices to walk in love. 1 John 4:16 says that 'God is love and he who abides in love abides in God, and God in him'. Amos 3:3 says 'can two walk together, unless they are agreed'. God is love and if we want to walk with him and have His presence and, by association, His power on our lives then we must walk in love. Offense, unforgiveness, strife, anger and other bad attitudes will remove the anointing from our lives.

3. Be obedient and faithful with what God has asked you to do

1 Peter 4:10

As each one has received a gift, minister it to one another, as good stewards of the manifold grace of God.

In the parable of the talents in Matthew 25:14-30 Jesus makes it clear that we are expected to serve Him with the talents that He gives each one and, as we do this faithfully, He will give us more. The scripture in 1 Peter 4:10 shows us that each gift is a measure of the grace of God, or His power by the Holy Spirit, upon our lives. Therefore, if we are faithful and receive more of His grace, then we will, by association, have more of His power on us.

4. Pursue the presence of God through prayer

Many a time in Jesus' ministry, He drew aside on His own to pray to His heavenly Father. He made time for the Father. In the midst of a busy ministry, He didn't think that He didn't have time to pray. In Acts 6:4, the apostles make the wise decision that 'we will give ourselves continually to prayer and the ministry of the word'.

There is no power without prayer. Prayer is not primarily presenting requests to God, although He does respond to this. Prayer is seeking God Himself, with the intent to know Him and encounter His presence. In His presence, His power will come upon you.

This is not something that can be accomplished by trying to squeeze prayer into our busy lives wherever it may fit. Prayer has to be the priority. Often when people come for pastoral advice, the first question is 'How is your prayer life?' Too many times the answer is 'a quick prayer in the car or train on the way to work'. That would be fine if it was in addition to your main prayer time but on its own is not enough. People are astounded when they see how much their circumstances start to turn around, as they prioritise prayer and don't just slot it in somewhere. We need to put the seeking of God's presence, and not just His blessing, as top priority if we want to have His anointing.

Before Jesus, the only access into the presence of God, beyond the veil into the Holy of Holies in the temple, was by the High Priest once a year as he made atonement for the sins of the people. The physical pathway that the priest took into the presence of God in the Old Testament is a pattern for how we enter into God's presence spiritually in the New Testament. I am going to outline a strategy that I often use in my own prayer time to enter into the presence of God. Unlike the Old Testament saints, we can be in His presence every day of our lives.

Hebrews 9:6 -10
Now when these things had been thus prepared, the priests always went into the first part of the tabernacle, performing the services. But into the second part the high priest went alone once a year, not without blood, which he offered for himself and for the people's sins committed in ignorance; the Holy Spirit indicating this, that the way into the Holiest of All was not yet made manifest while the first tabernacle was still standing. It was symbolic for the present time in which both gifts and sacrifices are offered which cannot make him who performed the service perfect in regard to the conscience— concerned only with foods and drinks, various washings, and fleshly ordinances imposed until the time of reformation.

The first thing that the priest would do is enter the gate into the tabernacle. The gate is a picture or symbol of Jesus. He is the door or the entrance into the presence of God and the Kingdom of God.

John 10:9, 10 Jesus speaking
"I am the door. If anyone enters by Me, he will be saved, and will go in and out and find pasture. The thief does not come except to

steal, and to kill, and to destroy. I have come that they may have life, and that they may have it more abundantly."

Next the High Priest would come to the altar where a sacrifice was made, the blood covering his sins. In the Old Testament the blood of an animal was shed and was seen to cover the sins of the people. That cover protected the people from judgment but it did not have the power to remove sin. It was also done in faith, looking forward to the time when sin would be paid for by Jesus' sacrifice. In His shed blood provision was also made for all the sins that had gone before, and the Old Testament saints who had exercised faith in God through their sacrifices had their sins completely removed then. That is why the Old Testament saints could not go up to heaven immediately, instead going to a place called Paradise until Jesus had come and paid for all their sins. Covering them was not enough to gain entry into Heaven. After Jesus' resurrection, the Old Testament saints were also raised and went to Heaven with Him at that time.

Matthew 27:51-53
Then, behold, the veil of the temple was torn in two from top to bottom; and the earth quaked, and the rocks were split, and the graves were opened; and many bodies of the saints who had fallen asleep were raised; and coming out of the graves after His resurrection, they went into the holy city and appeared to many.

In the New Testament, the blood of Jesus completely removes sin from us, thus allowing us to come into God's presence. Not only that, but His blood has the power to cleanse our conscience.

Hebrews 9:11-14
But Christ came as High Priest of the good things to come, with the greater and more perfect tabernacle not made with hands, that is, not of this creation. Not with the blood of goats and calves, but with His own blood He entered the Most Holy Place once for all, having obtained eternal redemption. For if the blood of bulls and goats and the ashes of a heifer, sprinkling the unclean, sanctifies

for the purifying of the flesh, how much more shall the blood of Christ, who through the eternal Spirit offered Himself without spot to God, cleanse your conscience from dead works to serve the living God?

The first key to entering the presence of God is to come through Jesus and to thank Him. So, you start by praising and thanking Him for all that He has done and for bringing you to the Father. I also go through many of the things that He has done for me in my personal walk with Him, all the miracles, healings and blessings. Psalm 100:4 says *'Enter into His gates with thanksgiving, and into His courts with praise. Be thankful to Him, and bless His name.'* Already you can feel God's presence just by doing this.

The High Priest would next come to the bronze laver where he would wash, symbolic of the cleansing by the Holy Spirit through repentance. When we are saved, we are cleansed from all sin but along the way we will sin again. Repentance from these actions, symbolized by the washing of the hands and feet, removes the stain of these sins.

Therefore, the second key into entering God's presence is repentance. Repent of any sins and ask for forgiveness and cleansing from anything that may have defiled you in your daily walk. Examples might be negative thinking, critical or unloving thoughts or words; anything that might separate you from God's presence.

The priest then entered the Holy Place. On one side was a table with the Showbread. Bread is symbolic of Jesus, the Bread of Life, and the Word of God (Matthew 4:4). On the other side was a lamp, with oil that had to burn continually. The lamp, also symbolic of the Word of God (Psalm 119:105), was made of one piece of gold that had 66 parts. Some say that if you take the centre parts that comprise the stand and the parts to the left, then you have 39 parts on one side and 27 on the other. The Bible has 66 books, 39 in the Old Testament and 27 in the New Testament. The oil throughout the Bible is symbolic of the Holy Spirit. The oil in the lamp had to burn continually, symbolizing the need for revelation that comes with the Holy Spirit inspiring the Word of God to us.

We are not to read the Bible, the Word of God, as some dry list of rules and regulations. We need to pray for the Holy Spirit to reveal it to our spirits. You find that as you are reading the Bible, passages 'come alive' to you; you receive inner understanding and see how it applies to your life or are inspired to change in line with it. This is the revelation that comes from the Holy Spirit. It is this that brings faith into your spirit (Romans 10:17). Reading the Bible is so important but if you just read it without the inspiration of the Holy Spirit, it is not necessarily bringing faith. The oil of the Holy Spirit has to burn continually on the Word of God.

The third key, then, is reading the Word of God and speaking it out over your life. Faith comes by hearing and hearing, not just reading. As the Holy Spirit gives you 'rhemas' over the years, speak them out in your prayer time and speak out any promises of God that you need for your life. Faith is coming as you do this. Therefore, before you even ask God for anything, you have glorified Him and reminded yourself of how great He is, repented from any blockages between yourself and Him and built up your spirit in faith.

Now when you pray you are not approaching God timidly, wondering if He will do or even is able to do what you are asking, but you are confident in Who He is and approaching Him in faith. This is so important because all that we receive from God is through our faith in Him and not just as a response to our need.

Hebrews 11:6

But without faith it is impossible to please Him, for he who comes to God must believe that He is, and that He is a rewarder of those who diligently seek Him.

Romans 4:16

Therefore it is of faith that it might be according to grace, so that the promise might be sure to all the seed, not only to those who are of the law, but also to those who are of the faith of Abraham, who is the father of us all.

The priest then came to an altar where he offered up incense before going through a veil into the Holy of Holies, where the presence of God dwelt. The Bible says that our prayers go up before God as incense (Revelation 5:8, 8:3). Prayer and worship bring you into the presence of God. At this point, you start to offer up your prayers, now doing this from a position of faith, and you worship God for Himself and the expected answers.

Finally the priest would enter through a thick veil (that kept the people separated from God's presence) into the Holy of Holies where God's presence was. That veil was torn from top to bottom the instant that Jesus died on the Cross. He made the way open into the presence of God!

In the Holy of Holies was the Ark of the Covenant, containing the Ten Commandments, some of the manna that the Hebrews had lived on in the wilderness for forty years, and the rod of the high priest, Aaron, that God had miraculously budded. In the presence of God is revelation of His will and Word, understanding of His ways and our way, spiritual food that sustains us through all seasons, and miracles.

The last key to entering God's presence is to wait upon Him after going through all the other steps. In that place you find all the richness of your relationship with Him, direction and wisdom, and miracles start to happen in your life. Too many people want the quick fix, the speedy miracle based on the quick prayer time that fits in with a busy life. It doesn't happen that way. It takes time to get into that place with God and then to wait upon Him for His leading, understanding and empowerment. I find that miracles are a by-product of seeking God for Himself. The more that I focus on Him and being in His presence, the more miracles just happen and answers to prayer come more easily.

Isaiah 40:31
But those who wait on the Lord shall renew their strength; They shall mount up with wings like eagles, they shall run and not be weary, They shall walk and not faint.

As you take time to wait upon God, you exchange your strength for His, your questions for His answers and your needs for His power and miracles. It is also as we just sit in His presence that we receive His empowerment which is His anointing.

So we:
1. **Spend time thanking and praising God**
2. **Repent from any sin**
3. **Speak out the Word of God to bring faith**
4. **Prayer and worship**
5. **Wait on God in His presence**

In addition to your daily prayer, times of fasting with prayer bring the presence of God in a far greater manner than prayer alone. After times of fasting combined with increased periods of prayer, you find that you have more of the presence of God, pray more powerfully and speak the Word of God more boldly and the anointing is greatly increased.

Matthew 9:14, 15
Then the disciples of John came to him, saying, "Why do we and the Pharisees fast often, but Your disciples do not fast?"

And Jesus said to them, "Can the friends of the bridegroom mourn as long as the bridegroom is with them? But the days will come when the bridegroom will be taken away from them, and then they will fast".

The disciples didn't need to fast while Jesus was so close to them. However, when He went to Heaven, then they would need to fast to draw near to Him. Fasting brings us closer to God, as we are desperate for His presence, and, in so doing, the anointing will increase.

5. Meditate on the word; build up your faith
Jesus was the Word of God made flesh. We have to allow the Word of God to be made flesh in us if we are to live and minister the way that Jesus did.

We must have the Word abiding in us. We do this by studying it, meditating on it, allowing the Holy Spirit to illuminate it, and then acting on it in order for this to happen.

John 8:31, 32

If you abide in My word, you are My disciples indeed. And you shall know the truth, and the truth shall make you free.

Jesus' words are spirit, as He is, and as we receive them and allow them to become flesh in us (that is, allow His truth to change us) they bring His life and His Spirit into us. With His life and Spirit is His power.

John 6:63

It is the Spirit Who gives life; the flesh profits nothing. The words that I speak to you are spirit and life.

The Word of God brings faith (Romans 10:17) and the Holy Spirit is always attracted to faith. Right from the time of Creation, the Holy Spirit has moved on the Word of God spoken in faith.

So we need to;
1. Pursue holiness and overcome sin
2. Be obedient and faithful with what God has asked us to do
3. Walk in love
4. Keep prayer as a priority
5. Meditate on the word

If we decrease in these areas, then the anointing on our life will then decrease due to:
1. Lack of holiness or sin grieving the Holy Spirit
2. Disobedience removing us from God's path and unfaithfulness resulting in our talents being given to another.
3. Not walking in love grieves the Holy Spirit.
4. No presence and hence, no power, if there is no prayer.
5. Unbelief because our Word life is down.

Over time you will develop an awareness of the anointing of the Holy Spirit for healing. Everyone feels the anointing differently but I feel it as a presence moving down my right arm and what feels like a ball of heat in the palm of my hands, usually the right hand but sometimes both. When that comes, I know that the presence of the Lord is there to heal. If I don't feel anything, then I pray according to the prayer of faith that whatever I ask when I pray I believe that I receive it and I shall have it.

PICTURE

SEE YOURSELF AS SET APART FOR GOD AND CARRYING THE PRESENCE OF THE HOLY SPIRIT-

THEN YOU WILL WALK AND MAKE LIFE CHOICES IN LINE WITH HOW YOU SEE YOURSELF.

THE MEANS OF MINISTERING HEALING

There are many ways that the anointing can be transferred from one believer to another. I am going to discuss only four of these; the laying on of hands, anointing with oil, through the spoken word and, when necessary, through deliverance. There are also the gifts of healings and miracles that the Spirit gives as He wills, as revealed in 1 Corinthians 12, but I am going to just share on those aspects of ministry that all can be involved in.

THE LAYING ON OF HANDS

Hebrews 6:1, 2
Therefore, leaving the discussion of the elementary principles of Christ, let us go on to perfection, not laying again the foundation of repentance from dead works and of faith toward God, of the doctrine of baptisms, of laying on of hands, of resurrection of the dead, and of eternal judgment.

The laying on of hands is one of the basic doctrines of God, used in both the Old and New Testaments, as a means to impart a gift or transfer the anointing from one person to another.

One example in the Old Testament is where God had anointed Moses with wisdom. So this was not a natural human wisdom but a God-empowered, supernatural wisdom, so that he could solve the problems of the people who came to him for help.

Numbers 27 records the transference of leadership to Joshua as Moses' death approaches and Deuteronomy 34 records the death of Moses, with verse nine revealing that the same power that had been on Moses to lead the people had been transferred to Joshua through the laying on of hands.

Numbers 27:18-20
And the Lord said to Moses: "Take Joshua the son of Nun with you, a man in whom is the Spirit, and lay your hand on him; set him before Eleazar the priest and before all the congregation, and inaugurate him in their sight. And you shall give some of your authority to him, that all the congregation of the children of Israel may be obedient.

Deuteronomy 34:9
Now Joshua the son of Nun was full of the spirit of wisdom, for Moses had laid his hands on him; so the children of Israel heeded him, and did as the Lord had commanded Moses.

Jesus and then his disciples ministered healing often through the laying on of hands, transferring the anointing that was on them to the sick person. In Acts 19:6, Paul lays hands on believers to receive the Holy Spirit, transferring the anointing or power of the Holy Spirit that was upon him (from being filled with the Holy Spirit) to those who had not yet received Him.

In Mark 16:15-18, Jesus is giving His final words to, not only His disciples, but to all those who believe in Him, which includes His present day disciples. Recall that He had already said that those who believed in Him would do the works that He did and even greater works (John 14:12). He tells us that these believers will lay hands on the sick and they will recover. The laying on of hands was to be one of the main means by which we would do His works, transferring His healing power from the believer to those who need healing. Again, this promise is not restricted to those in recognised positions of ministry or leadership. The promise is to all who choose to walk as a disciple of Jesus, abiding in His Word and living it.

Mark 16: 15 -18

And He said to them, "Go into all the world and preach the gospel to every creature. He who believes and is baptized will be saved; but he who does not believe will be condemned. And these signs will follow those who believe: In My name they will cast out demons; they will speak with new tongues; they will take up serpents; and if they drink anything deadly, it will by no means hurt them; they will lay hands on the sick, and they will recover."

In addition to Jesus' ongoing will for the sick to be healed, healing in this context also reveals the importance of healings and miracles in presenting the gospel. The power of God revealed in a way that demonstrates His love and concern for people opens their hearts to hear the message. It is the goodness of God that leads people to repentance.

Those not yet saved are not healed through the believing of the Word but, rather as a miracle, demonstrating God's reality and goodness. However, for believers faith is required most of the time. There are occasions where people are healed on an altar call or through the prayer of others, without faith, but this is not meant to be the rule of thumb. The gospels reveal that about half of the healings Jesus performed were through the anointing being transferred to a person of faith, which tells me that faith is crucial for the believer to receive most of the time.

Now it is important to remember that healing is ministered through faith and received through faith. Romans 10:17 says that *'faith comes by hearing and hearing by the word of God'*. Faith comes. That tells me that it is not always there. Before praying for people, we need to make sure that our own faith is built up, that we are someone who actively believes, and that we take time to help the person being healed to be positioned in faith.

```
           God's blessings on
              the path        → Pressure from the devil
           -given by grace    - doubt, deception and
                                discouragement to get
                                you out of faith
                              → temptation to get you
                                into disobedience and
                                off the path
Position yourself
on the path by                        Promises
Faith and                          received through
Obedience        ───────→  ←───────  Faith
```

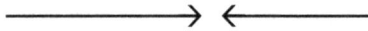

We need to be encouraging people to believe God for their healing so that they are in alignment to receive His blessing of healing. We also need to be aware that they will be bombarded with doubt, deception and discouragement and we need to be counteracting that. Share the scriptures on healing with the person; address any deceptions, particularly religious teachings that have told them that healing is not for all or that somehow God may not heal them. Also, since healing is usually a process and not instantaneous, keep encouraging them to stay in faith and not to be discouraged if things don't change straight away. Even though personal testimonies are encouraging, don't restrict your sharing to them alone. People need the Word of God to have faith.

The first person that I prayed for to be healed was when I was a young believer, knowing a few scriptures but really not knowing much. The gentleman that I prayed for had a haemorrhaging stomach ulcer. I went to him and just shared those few scriptures that I knew until he understood them. I then prayed a very simple prayer, not knowing any other type at the time. That gentleman was instantly healed, not only from the haemorrhaging but completely from having the ulcer. He was in church a few days later, completely well. That tells me that you don't have to know everything and you don't need to be a 'someone'. You just need the Word of God in you, and shared with the sick person, bringing faith on both sides.

How to pray for someone, with the laying on of hands.
I find it helpful to keep in mind the four steps of faith that I outlined in 'Receiving healing by faith'.

1. Believe or attend to the Word
2. Believe in your heart
3. Speak out the Word
4. Act in faith

Before praying, it is good to ascertain where the person is regarding their faith.

1. Believe or attend to the Word
Always encourage the person that God is their Healer, that He is full of mercy and willing to heal them; that Jesus has already borne this sickness on their behalf and that it can be removed in the same way as sin is removed from us when we receive forgiveness; and that nothing is impossible with God. Have scriptures memorised that you can share with them, and explain the gospel of healing to them.

When finding out what they need healing for and where they are at, it is good to not let them go into lengthy detail about their condition. This is not lack of compassion but actually an important factor in the positioning in faith. If you allow the person to go on and on about the problem their faith is going down, and often, so is yours. Unbelief on either side stops the anointing of healing flowing. Remember, God knows all the details of what they have and what needs to be done and so, for the sake of the minister and the person being healed, it's best to get the edited version.

Where possible, I find it best to not pray until I know the person is in faith. If you just rush in and pray without positioning them in faith then they are less likely to be healed, resulting in discouragement or doubt that healing is for them. In Jesus' ministry often the person came with a statement of belief before He would pray. In the absence of this, He asked in Matthew 9:28, *"Do you believe that I am able to do this?"*. In verse 29, He says, *"According to your faith let it be to you"*. In Luke 8:50, after Jairus receives the discouraging news that his daughter has just died, Jesus says to him, *"Do not be afraid; only believe and she will be made well"*.

2. Believe in your heart

I ask the person to see themself healed, or doing something that they couldn't do before, so that they are positioned in faith. Then, as I lay my hand on them, I either visualise them being healed, or more usually, I see an image of Jesus suffering on the Cross, that I carry in my heart. I see Him carrying the person's affliction, suffering it on their behalf, thereby bringing their healing to them. I find that a better focus for my faith than trying to see the healing of another, especially if I don't know the person.

Before laying hands on someone, I ask them if they are comfortable with me doing so, and then, make sure that it is done in a way that cannot cause offence or discomfort.

3. Speak out the Word

In the name of Jesus, declare the Word of God over the person, command the sickness to go using the authority that Jesus has given you in His Name.

Don't ask God to do the healing for you. He has told us to heal the sick in His name. Not for a moment do you think that the healing comes from you but be confident in the authority He has given you and His power that He has entrusted in you to do what is His Will.

4. Act in faith

Encourage the person to keep thanking God that they have received their healing, until it fully manifests.

Don't be concerned as to whether the person falls under the power of the Spirit or not. Sometimes people fall but are not healed. At other times, they stand there without much response, and they are healed. Falling under the power of the Spirit is a valid response to encountering the power of God, through the anointing on the minister, or in the atmosphere of a meeting. However, the receiving of healing has more to do with the response of faith to that anointing and the power of God's Word.

I often pray for a plan of healing for a person. Jesus said of His own ministry that He only did what He saw the Father do (John 5:19). We should only do what we see Jesus do. An example of such a plan that He has given me is in John 11 with Jesus raising Lazarus from the dead.

Firstly in John 11:39, He says to take away the stone. The analogy is to remove all unbelief and hardness of heart through encouraging the person to believe. Then Jesus gives the 'rhema' for the situation in verse 40. This is the scripture that I apply my faith to.

John 11:40
Jesus said to her, "Did I not say to you that if you would believe you would see the glory of God".

Then you call forth the life and healing that Jesus has provided, as He calls Lazarus forth in verse 43. Finally, loose the person from any spirit of infirmity or anything that has kept them in bondage to that sickness, as Jesus commands Lazarus to be loosed.

Jesus spent long hours in prayer before praying for the sick, receiving God's power and in that place, I believe, seeing what His Father did. We too find the power to pray and the strategy to release healing in our private prayer time. All the breaking through of hindrances, receiving of promises through faith, taking hold of the kingdom and dealing with demonic hindrances is done beforehand in your prayer time.

Once equipped and empowered, then you go and pray for the person, at which time only a simple prayer is required to release what you have already laid hold of. We should not be doing long prayers, shouting at the devil or any weird behaviour in ministering, especially in places, such as hospitals, where not all are believers. Do all long prayers, fighting of faith and taking authority over the devil in private. The release of the healing or breakthrough publically is simple, short, authoritative and never weird.

PICTURE

SEE THE PERSON BEING HEALED OR SEE JESUS BEARING THEIR SICKNESS OR AFFLICTION FOR THEM, AS YOU ARE PRAYING.

THE ANOINTING WITH OIL

James 5:14, 15

Is anyone among you sick? Let him call for the elders of the church, and let them pray over him, anointing him with oil in the name of the Lord. And the prayer of faith will save the sick, and the Lord will raise him up. And if he has committed sins, he will be forgiven.

Mark 6:13

And they cast out many demons, and anointed with oil many who were sick, and healed them.

I would use this mainly in the area of serious illness, for those in hospital or for those who find it hard to believe, but it is certainly not restricted to that. Now it is important to recognise that the oil has no healing properties but is symbolic of the Holy Spirit. I once had a lady from another denomination come to me for prayer for healing for her daughter. She had erroneously been told by their minister that healing in Biblical times came through a special oil that was used at that time and, as we no longer have access to that oil, then healing was no longer available. Any oil can be used, as it is a symbol and not the healer.

As discussed in 'Receiving healing through Communion', sometimes more power is released when we use the symbols, the person's faith having a contact point and God responding as if it really were the Holy Spirit being put on them. Also, in context with the discussion on the anointing, the anointing can be stored in a person or even things, such as cloths. Hence, the oil can store the anointing of the person praying and allow that anointing to abide on the sick person.

Now James says that the prayer of faith will save or heal the sick, that prayer being offered by the elder. Usually when this prayer is offered, the person receiving healing is not in a state to believe for themselves. Therefore, in such cases, I would make a commitment to stand in faith for that person, until they are healed, which is not something you can feasibly do for every person that you pray for. So, I believe for them using the prayer of faith according to Jesus in Mark 11:24 and based on the truth of healing in the scriptures. You believe when you pray, whether there is a physical manifestation at that time or not, and trust that it will be done as you continue to stand in faith.

Mark 11:24
Therefore I say to you, whatever things you ask when you pray, believe that you receive them, and you will have them.

If possible, I would use the steps of faith as outlined in the section on the laying on of hands. However, if the person is really unwell, you may not be able to encourage them to believe or see themselves well. So, I see Jesus bearing their sickness, apply the oil to their forehead seeing the Holy Spirit bringing His healing power. Then I speak the Word of God over them and command the sickness to leave and for them to be filled with the healing power that Jesus has provided for them, through the Holy Spirit, represented by the oil.

PICTURE

SEE THE PERSON HEALED, JESUS BEARING THEIR SICKNESS AND REMOVING IT FROM THEM AND THE HOLY SPIRIT COMING ON THEM WITH THE APPLIED OIL.

HEALING THROUGH
SPEAKING THE WORD

Psalm 107:20
He sent His word and healed them, and delivered them from their destructions.

God's Word contains His life, presence and power to bring healing. When released, we are healed. In the beginning, God created the heavens, the earth and all that it is in them by His spoken Word.

Hebrews 11:3
By faith we understand that the worlds were framed by the Word of God, so that the things which are seen were not made out of things which were visible.

God then created man in His own image and the words that we also speak are a creative or destructive force, bringing blessing or cursing. Proverbs 18:21 says that we will see fruit or results from our words, whatever they may be. God's Word in our mouths brings God's results.

Proverbs 18:21
Death and life are in the power of the tongue and those who love it will eat its fruit.

In Matthew 8, a Roman Centurion comes to Jesus, demonstrating the understanding that a word from Him is enough for a healing to take place, and in this case, without the sick person even being present. Jesus celebrates this Centurion's faith that allows a healing to take place this way, revealing that the spoken Word is sufficient to transfer the healing power of God.

Matthew 8:5-13

Now when Jesus had entered Capernaum, a centurion came to Him, pleading with Him, saying, "Lord, my servant is lying at home paralyzed, dreadfully tormented."

And Jesus said to him, "I will come and heal him."

The centurion answered and said, "Lord, I am not worthy that You should come under my roof. But only speak a word, and my servant will be healed. For I also am a man under authority, having soldiers under me. And I say to this one, 'Go,' and he goes; and to another, 'Come,' and he comes; and to my servant, 'Do this,' and he does it."

When Jesus heard it, He marveled, and said to those who followed, "Assuredly, I say to you, I have not found such great faith, not even in Israel! And I say to you that many will come from east and west, and sit down with Abraham, Isaac, and Jacob in the kingdom of heaven. But the sons of the kingdom will be cast out into outer darkness. There will be weeping and gnashing of teeth." Then Jesus said to the centurion, "Go your way; and as you have believed, so let it be done for you." And his servant was healed that same hour.

The centurion understood how authority works and that Jesus' word carried the power of the One who had delegated authority to Him. Under the Roman government the centurion had been given authority and when he spoke it carried the power of the government he served. He understood that Jesus was operating under God's authority and that everything else was under His authority. When He spoke it carried the power of God, the One who had given Him that authority.

In the same way, the authority we operate in, when we minister, comes from Jesus and operates in His Name. When we position ourselves under Him in obedience and faith, and operate according to His Word and will, then, when we speak, it carries the power of God (who gave us His authority).

In Acts 14 we see Paul speaking a word to release God's healing anointing. What is important to notice is that Paul first waited to see that faith was present, watching the man intently before doing this. This indicates to me that a higher level of faith is required in the person receiving healing for it to be ministered this way.

Acts 14:8-10

And in Lystra a certain man without strength in his feet was sitting, a cripple from his mother's womb, who had never walked. This man heard Paul speaking. Paul, observing him intently and seeing that he had faith to be healed, said with a loud voice, "Stand up straight on your feet!" And he leaped and walked.

Romans 10:8-10

But what does it say? "The word is near you, in your mouth and in your heart" (that is, the word of faith which we preach):that if you confess with your mouth the Lord Jesus and believe in your heart that God has raised Him from the dead, you will be saved. For with the heart one believes unto righteousness, and with the mouth confession is made unto salvation.

If the Word is spoken in combination with a believing heart then we can be saved. The word saved here is 'sozo' meaning, not only to save, but to heal and be made whole. So, we can declare the Word by faith and release healing into our bodies and those we are praying for. Then Jeremiah 1:12 reveals that God is watching over His Word to fulfil it and Isaiah 55:11 that His Word, spoken by Him but, also by us, will accomplish His will.

Mark 16:20

And they went out and preached everywhere, the Lord working with them and confirming the word through the accompanying signs. Amen.

Jeremiah 1:12 NIV
The LORD said to me, "You have seen correctly, for I am watching to see that my word is fulfilled."[7]

Isaiah 55:11
So shall My word be that goes forth from My mouth; it shall not return to Me void, but it shall accomplish what I please, And it shall prosper in the thing for which I sent it.

Examples in Scripture

Matthew 9:6,7 Jesus heals the paralytic (Mk 2:10,11,Lk 17-25)
...then He said to the paralytic, "Arise, take up your bed, and go to your house." And he arose and departed to his house.

Luke 7:12 -15 Raising from the dead the son of the widow of Nain
Then He came and touched the open coffin, and those who carried him stood still. And He said, "Young man, I say to you, arise." So he who was dead sat up and began to speak. And He presented him to his mother.

John 11:43, 44 Raising Lazarus from the dead
Now when He had said these things, He cried with a loud voice, "Lazarus, come forth!" And he who had died came out bound hand and foot with graveclothes, and his face was wrapped with a cloth. Jesus said to them, "Loose him, and let him go."

John 5:8, 9 Man healed at the pool of Bethesda
Jesus said to him, "Rise, take up your bed and walk." And immediately the man was made well, took up his bed, and walked. And that day was the Sabbath.

Acts 9:33, 34 Peter heals Aeneas
There he found a certain man named Aeneas, who had been bedridden eight years and was paralyzed. And Peter said to him, "Aeneas, Jesus the Christ heals you. Arise and make your bed." Then he arose immediately.

Acts 9:40, 41 Peter raises Dorcas from the dead

But Peter put them all out, and knelt down and prayed. And turning to the body he said, "Tabitha, arise." And she opened her eyes, and when she saw Peter she sat up. Then he gave her his hand and lifted her up; and when he had called the saints and widows, he presented her alive.

PICTURE

GOD SEES HIS WORD BEING FULFILLED- WE NEED TO SEE THE SAME THING!

HEALING THROUGH DELIVERANCE

There are occasions when a sickness or affliction may be the effect of a demonic spirit or, a spirit of infirmity that needs to be removed for healing to come. There are many times in Jesus' ministry where He did not lay his hands on a person or speak a word but, instead, cast out a spirit. In reading about such healings, it is important not to assume that every time a person has the same condition that it must be due to a spirit.

Deliverance is not usually the first line of approach but would be considered after discussion with the person revealed the probability of a demonic presence, or the leading of the Holy Spirit indicates that to be the case. In such a case, there a few steps I would follow.

The first is to establish that the person is agreeable for you to pray this way. Even God will not operate against a person's will and we should not think that we can cast out a spirit unless the person's will is in line with this. Once they agree, I ask them to repent of the sin that allowed the devil to come in in the first place. This may not always be an obvious thing to them and so you may need to talk about their involvement in past spiritual activities, any areas of hate, anger or unforgiveness or drug and alcohol abuse. For many that I have prayed for, the entry point has been past visits to psychics, tarot card readers, palm readers or involvement in spiritualism or other religions. More often than not, people are surprised that this would have such an impact on them. What seemed like an innocent bit of fun going to a psychic opened the door for an evil presence and sickness in their life.

Following repentance, I pray the power of the blood of Jesus over them, the blood that has already destroyed all the powers of darkness. Then I command the spirit to leave them in the name of Jesus. Having done the previous steps, the actual deliverance usually takes place without too much resistance because the demon's power has been broken over that life. If not, persist until it leaves.

An example of this is when a lady came to me, having persistent difficulty in breathing, tightness in the chest and she was hunched over. Discussion revealed that she had backslidden at one point in her Christian walk and experimented with Buddhism and some of its spiritual practices. I lead her in a prayer of repentance, prayed the blood of Jesus over her and commanded any spirit that had entered her life through that experience to leave. Immediately, she drew in a deep breath and straightened up. She then described the feeling of huge talons being withdrawn from her back and lungs and a heavy weight released from her. She was completely healed.

We have been given authority by Jesus to cast out demons.

Luke 10:19
Behold, I give you the authority to trample on serpents and scorpions, and over all the power of the enemy, and nothing shall by any means hurt you.

Mark 16:17
And these signs will follow those who believe: In My name they will cast out demons; they will speak with new tongues;

Examples of healing through deliverance

Matthew 9:32, 33
As they went out, behold, they brought to Him a man, mute and demon-possessed. And when the demon was cast out, the mute spoke. And the multitudes marveled, saying, "It was never seen like this in Israel!"

Matthew 17: 14, 15, 18 (Mark 9:17-27- describes it as a deaf and dumb spirit)

And when they had come to the multitude, a man came to Him, kneeling down to Him and saying, "Lord, have mercy on my son, for he is an epileptic and suffers severely; for he often falls into the fire and often into the water........

And Jesus rebuked the demon, and it came out of him; and the child was cured from that very hour.

PICTURE

SEE YOUR AUTHORITY OVER THE DEVIL AND WHEN YOU COMMAND A SPIRIT TO GO, IT MUST LEAVE.

8

THE HEALING OF THE SOUL

....

3 John 2
Beloved, I pray that you may prosper in all things and be in health, just as your soul prospers.

John says that we are in health according to how our soul prospers. Sometimes, due to life's challenges, abuse, stress, unforgiveness or sin, the soul, which is our mind, will and emotions is not prospering. This can interfere with healing coming to the body.

God will still heal the person, but often the healing first needs to take place in the soul. I used to wonder, as I read the gospels, why the writer would say that Jesus healed every kind of sickness and every kind of disease. Weren't sickness and disease the same thing?

In our modern language, sickness and disease are used interchangeably. An old, but no longer used, meaning of the word disease was dis-ease. One of the meanings of the prefix 'dis', according to the Macquarie dictionary is a 'negative or opposing force'[12]. Disease could then be interpreted as a negative or opposing force to ease, or peace.

Perhaps Jesus' disciples were observing that, in addition to healing the sick, Jesus healed those with conditions characterised by a lack of peace. This is long before modern psychiatry or psychology were around to name certain conditions of the soul. The disciples were just seeing a lack of peace.

Jesus has provided healing for our souls just as much as for our spirits or bodies. God wants us whole in every area; spirit, soul and body.

1 Thessalonians 5:23

Now may the God of peace Himself sanctify you <u>completely</u>; and may your whole spirit, soul and body be preserved blameless at the coming of our Lord Jesus Christ.

Luke 4:18-19

"The Spirit of the LORD is upon Me, because He has anointed Me to preach the gospel to the poor; He has sent Me to heal the brokenhearted, to proclaim liberty to the captives and recovery of sight to the blind, to set at liberty those who are oppressed; to proclaim the acceptable year of the LORD."

Matt 11:28-30

"Come to me, all you who are weary and burdened, and I will give you rest. Take my yoke upon you and learn from me, for I am gentle and humble in heart, and you will find rest for your souls. For my yoke is easy and my burden is light."

Psalm 23:1-3

The LORD is my shepherd; I shall not want. He makes me to lie down in green pastures;
    He leads me beside the still waters. <u>He restores my soul</u>;

Isaiah 53:5

The chastisement of our peace was upon Him and by his stripes we are healed.

Isaiah 53 is the passage talking about Jesus bearing our sin and sickness, bringing healing to us. The price of bringing us peace, which I believe was by bearing our 'dis-ease' as well as sickness, was borne by Jesus on the Cross. Jesus restores peace to your soul. He has provided in His redemption for you to be redeemed and, if necessary healed, from fear, anxiety, depression and anything else that keeps you from enjoying peace.

Receiving healing for the soul

We receive healing for the soul in a very similar way to receiving healing for the body. We will see in the next chapter on how to remove any sin or unforgiveness which may be an issue in the suffering of the soul. Then we attend the Word of God on, not only healing scriptures but also scriptures on receiving God's divine peace, joy and His amazing love for us. We believe them in our heart, seeing ourselves the way God sees us, and with His promised peace and joy. We speak the scriptures out and, as we do, over time, the soul transforms to experience the fruit of the Spirit.

Galatians 5:22, 23

But the fruit of the Spirit is love, joy, peace, longsuffering, kindness, goodness, faithfulness, gentleness and self control.

James 1:21-22

Therefore lay aside all filthiness and overflow of wickedness, and receive with meekness the implanted word, which is able to save your souls.

The word 'save' is translated from the Greek, 'sozo,' which we now know can also be translated as 'heal'. James says we are to remove sin, receive the implanted word, which we have already discussed in 'Receiving healing by faith' and God's word has the power to heal your soul in the same way as to heal the body. The following are a few scriptures that will help in this area.

Romans 15:13

Now may the God of hope fill you with all joy and peace in believing, that you may abound in hope by the power of the Holy Spirit.

Nehemiah 8:10

...Do not sorrow. For the joy of the Lord is your strength.

Philippians 4:6, 7

Be anxious for nothing, but in everything by prayer and

supplication, with thanksgiving, let your requests be made known to God; and the peace of God, which surpasses all understanding, will guard your hearts and minds through Christ Jesus.

John 14:27
Peace I leave with you, My peace I give to you; not as the world gives do I give to you. Let not your heart be troubled, neither let it be afraid.

John 16:33
These things I have spoken to you, that in Me you may have peace. In the world you will have tribulation; but be of good cheer, I have overcome the world."

1 John 4:18, 19
There is no fear in love; but perfect love casts out fear, because fear involves torment. But he who fears has not been made perfect in love. We love Him because He first loved us.

2 Timothy 1:7
For God has not given us a spirit of fear, but of power and of love and of a sound mind.

PICTURE

SEE YOURSELF AS BEING FILLED WITH THE FRUIT OF THE SPIRIT.

YOU ARE A LOVING PERSON, FULL OF PEACE AND JOY. YOU ARE PATIENT AND KIND.

9

THE HINDRANCE OF SIN, ESPECIALLY UNFORGIVENESS

As discussed in the chapter, 'How sickness came to mankind', sin separates us from God, and by so doing, His promises. If we have sin in our lives that we are not dealing with or, find too hard to deal with, it can hinder us receiving healing. It doesn't have to remain that way. Every sin can be dealt with by the power of God working in our lives.

> God's blessings on
> the path
> -given by grace
> -forgiveness
> -healing
> -His promises

You position yourself
on the path by faith
and obedience ⎯⎯⎯⎯⎯⎯→

We are removed from that path of God's blessings and promises, that is, being in His will, by anything that shifts us out of faith or obedience. Sin not only separates us from God, but removes us out of His will and the receiving of His promises. Repentance and faith in Jesus' work of salvation, accomplished in His death and resurrection puts us back on the path.

However we don't want to stay in a place where we sin and just repent of it. We want to be able to rise above areas of sin, weakness or hindrances in our life.

Sin literally means to 'miss the mark', to miss what God had intended for us to be and to do. It's like you have a target in front of you and God says, that the right to have a relationship with Him and the entrance into Heaven comes with a perfect bullseye. If you live a life that is perfect in every way, in thought, attitude and action, then you have made the mark.

Apart from Jesus, none of us have been able to do this. You might say, "Well, I have lived a good life; I've kept the Ten Commandments; I don't hurt anyone". That's great but you would still not be perfect and, hence, still be off that bullseye. You might have missed the bullseye by a little or be way off the board but, the fact is, we have all missed it. That's why we needed a Saviour to make the way for us to have a right relationship with God and be able to go to Heaven.

In His mercy, God sent His perfect Son, Jesus, to earth. He lived a perfect life in every way. He then chose to take upon Himself all of our sins and, by association, all of our judgment that was due to us, and suffer the penalty for it in our place. Romans 6:23 says *'the wages of sin is death'* and Jesus died in our place. He then rose from the dead, all sin having been paid for in the eyes of God.

When we receive Jesus into our heart, we receive forgiveness for all of our sins that we have ever committed and, in exchange, we are given Jesus' perfect record, His bullseye. So, now, we can have a relationship with God and we can go to Heaven. It's just that it is never by our own effort.

Ephesians 2:8, 9
For <u>by grace you have been saved</u> through faith, and that <u>not of yourselves; it is the gift of God, not of works</u>, lest anyone should boast.

Being 'born again'
Receiving Jesus' salvation is called, by Him, being 'born again'. This is Jesus' terminology, not a classification of a certain brand

of Christian. Irrespective of what denomination you belong to, if you have Jesus in your heart and you have a right relationship with God, then you are born again.

John 3:3-6

Jesus answered and said to him, "Most assuredly, I say to you, unless one is born again, he cannot <u>see</u> the kingdom of God."

Nicodemus said to Him, "How can a man be born when he is old? Can he enter a second time into his mother's womb and be born?"

Jesus answered, "Most assuredly, I say to you, unless one is born of water and the Spirit, he cannot <u>enter</u> the kingdom of God. That which is born of the flesh is flesh, and that which is born of the Spirit is spirit.

Our first birth, of water and the flesh, is our physical birth. Our second birth, or being born of the Spirit or 'born again' occurs when we receive Jesus and His forgiveness. Immediately, the Holy Spirit brings the life of God into our spirit, just as Adam had originally before he sinned, making it alive again. The separation caused by sin is removed and we are reconnected with God and the life that flows from Him. (John 3:6)

Jesus explains in John 3:3-6 that we cannot understand, or see(verse 3), nor enter (verse 5) the kingdom of God by our works, that is, by being a good person or doing the right thing alone, but by being spiritually reborn. Therefore, if Jesus says that we can't enter Heaven except by being 'born again', then it's obviously really important.

Three aspects of receiving Jesus:-

1. Repentance from all sin, removing the blockage between you and God.

2. Acknowledge that Jesus paid the full price for your sin and receive Him as your Saviour. As we enter into a relationship with God, known as a covenant, our sins are exchanged for Christ's righteousness, as God sees our sin placed on Christ at the Cross and then, sees Christ's righteousness credited to us. Christ's righteousness brings us right standing with God and eternal life.

In Christ, God chose to make a covenant with us where He says, 'I and all My resources are available to you, should you ever have need of it'. In exchange for our sins, He gives us His righteousness; in exchange for our sicknesses He gives us His healing; in exchange for the problems we experience in this life, He gives us His redemption and answers.

2 Corinthians 1:20
For all the promises of God in Him are Yes, and in Him Amen, to the glory of God through us.

In Christ, all the promises of God, that are attached to His covenant, His will, are given to us and in Him are amen; that is, they are guaranteed, because of what Christ did for us.

2 Peter 1:2-4
Grace and peace be multiplied to you in the knowledge of God and of Jesus our Lord, <u>as His divine power has given to us all things that pertain to life and godliness</u>, through the knowledge of Him who called us by glory and virtue, <u>by which have been given to us exceedingly great and precious promises, that through these you may become partakers of the divine nature</u>, having escaped the corruption that is in the world through lust.

The blood that seals this amazing covenant, is the blood of God Himself, Jesus, Who came in the flesh to sacrifice Himself on our behalf. The book of Hebrews tells us that not only was He the sacrifice to secure the covenant, but He rose from the dead to also become the mediator of that covenant.

Hebrews 7:22
By so much more Jesus has become a surety of a better covenant.

Hebrews 7:25
Therefore He is also able to save to the uttermost those who come to God through Him, since He always lives to make intercession for them.

Hebrews 8: 6

But now He has obtained a more excellent ministry, inasmuch as He is also Mediator of a better covenant, which was established on better promises.

Hebrews 9:26b -28

...but now, once at the end of the ages, he has appeared to put away sin by the sacrifice of Himself. And as it is appointed for men to die once and then the judgment, so Christ was offered once to bear the sins of many. To those who eagerly wait for Him he will appear a second time, apart from sin, for salvation.

If you have not already received Jesus to be your Lord and Saviour, pray this prayer to God.

"Dear God, I ask you to forgive me. I repent of all sin. I acknowledge that Jesus has paid the price for all my sins and I ask you, Lord Jesus, to come into my heart. I ask to be born again and to receive Your Holy Spirit."

If you have prayed this prayer for the first time or are rededicating your life to God, then please contact a Bible teaching church near you and speak to a pastor or other leader about how to live out this new life in Christ.

3. Receive Jesus as your **Lord** as well as your Saviour.

Romans 10:9

That if you confess with your mouth Jesus is Lord and believe in your heart that God raised Him from the dead, you will be saved.

The nature of the blood covenant is that it is a two way relationship. It is not enough to receive from God all of His incredible benefits and salvation and leave it at that. In response, we now say to Him, 'I and all my resources are available to you, should you ever have need of it'. This is a response of love and gratitude for all that He did for us.

2 Corinthians 5:14, 15

For the love of Christ compels us, because we judge thus: that if

One died for all, then all died; and He died for all, that those who live should no longer live for themselves, but for Him who died for them and rose again.

To do this, we need to understand repentance and then move beyond that, to living above the sin nature and live in the power of the Spirit.

Repentance

The day of your salvation, you receive a perfectly clean slate. How amazing! However, do we keep it that way? Do we go away from that moment of receiving Christ and live a perfect life? No. While choosing to live a changed life, we still go and daily add things onto that nice clean slate. Wrong thought patterns, wrong attitudes, being offended with people or acting out in a wrong way.

When we repent of these sins, God will wipe that slate clean again. We go to God and say, "I'm sorry, I blew it and I want to change in this area'. That is repentance, confessing your sin to God as well as making a decision to turn away from that sin. When we do that, God forgives us completely.

1 John 1:9
If we confess our sins, he is faithful and just to forgive us our sins and to cleanse us from all unrighteousness.

Jesus has already paid the price for every sin that you will ever commit. That does not mean that we ever intentionally sin, thinking that we can get away with it because God has forgiven us. If we are truly saved and experienced the change of heart that takes place, then we will not intentionally sin. Grace is never to be abused. Never forget the extraordinary cost that was paid for your, and my, forgiveness.

Proverbs 28:13
He who covers his sins will not prosper,
But whoever confesses and forsakes them will have mercy.

We are to both confess and forsake sin. If we cover our sins, thinking no one knows about that area in our life, it will stop us prospering, it can cause sickness or it can hinder us receiving healing. In John 5:14, after healing the man at the pool of Bethesda, a man who had the infirmity thirty-eight years, Jesus identifies sin as being the issue behind his suffering.

John 5:14
Afterward Jesus found him in the temple, and said to him, "See you have been made well. Sin no more, lest a worse thing come upon you."

Remember that 'law of sin and death' discussed in the chapter on 'How sickness came to mankind'?

immediate   ←   over a period of time   →

SIN → SPIRITUAL → SICKNESS & DISEASE → PHYSICAL

DEATH   HUMAN SUFFERING   DEATH

THE CURSE

← root cause →←fruit that came into the earth as a result→

If we choose to deliberately hang onto an area of sin and not let it go (this does not mean being perfect but willfully and unrepentantly sinning in a particular area), then the consequences of sin or exposure to the curse can come back into our life. It's a law - sin cannot be separated from its consequences. Galatians 6:8 says that *'he who sows to the flesh will of the flesh reap corruption.'* Hanging onto an area of sin can bring sickness or hinder the receiving of healing.

What if you have a sin that you can't deal with?
Sometimes when we read a scripture, we can feel "I cannot do this!" So, I am going to share a story with you of how God enables you to deal with areas of your life that you are just not able to deal with.

For years prior to receiving Christ, I knew that He was calling me. However, I also knew that if I became a Christian that there was someone in my past whom I would have to forgive. I reasoned that I was unable to forgive and therefore, would not become a Christian, because I don't do things in half measures.

If I was to be saved, then I would be 100% that way.

Let me emphasize to you here, that God never asked us to be perfect before coming to Him. That is impossible. He just asks us to come as we are, and He does the perfecting in our lives.

I eventually went to church and made the commitment to receive Christ. A very short time afterwards, a pastor got up to speak on forgiveness. I thought to myself, 'I knew it; I knew this was going to come; I can't do it'.

While not recalling what he literally said, he shared a story that brought out that God was asking you to be willing and obedient but not to be able. We were never meant to live God's way in our own strength. If we could do that, then we didn't need a Saviour.

God asks us to be willing to do things His way. Then we take a step of obedience in that direction but He provides the ability or grace to do it, by the power of His Holy Spirit.

I said, "Ok Lord, I am willing and I will choose to be obedient but to tell you the truth I have absolutely no ability in me to do this." Richard and I asked this person out to dinner and I made the step to reach out to them with reconciliation. As I made that step, I felt the love of God completely flood me, releasing me from all unforgiveness toward that person.

James 4:6 Amplified
But He gives us more and more grace (power of the Holy Spirit, to meet this evil tendency and all others fully). That is why He says, God sets Himself against the proud and haughty, but gives grace (continually) to the lowly (those who are humble enough to receive it).[3]

When we ask for God's help, He gives us His grace. The Amplified version here says that His grace is 'the power of the Holy Spirit to meet this evil tendency and all others fully'. In other words, God gives His power to you to overcome <u>any</u> sin <u>fully</u>. We just have to position ourselves to receive His help.

Now you might be struggling with a different issue. It might be anger, impatience, addictions or unclean thoughts. The principle to overcoming is exactly the same. Be willing and make steps of obedience to walk away from that sin, and God will give you His power to overcome.

I want to emphasize the importance of not carrying unforgiveness. In every class that I teach in our new Christian classes, I find that at least one person in a group will be struggling with this issue. If you haven't had to deal with it, stay around people long enough, and it will probably rear its ugly head.

Mark 11:25, 26

And whenever you stand praying, if you have anything against anyone, forgive him, that your Father in heaven may also forgive you your trespasses. But if you do not forgive, neither will your Father in heaven forgive your trespasses.

This is so important because Jesus says here if we don't forgive, then we won't receive God's forgiveness. If we are not positioned to receive His forgiveness then we are certainly not positioned to be healed. Not only that, but unforgiveness can be a source of sickness in the body, as the person constantly revisits the original offence with all of its associated trauma and chemical responses in the body. It needs to be removed before healing comes.

Overcoming sin to live in the power of the Spirit

We are saved by grace, through faith, and not by works but, once saved, James 2:17, 18 reveals that a genuine faith will reveal itself in good works. We need to make the choice to live in a way that is pleasing to God, being dead to the old nature of sin and rising to live in the new nature, empowered by the Holy Spirit and the Word of God, becoming who God has designed us to be.

2 Corinthians 5:17

Therefore, if anyone is in Christ, he is a new creation; old things have passed away; behold, all things have become new.

Romans 6:4-6

Therefore we were buried with him through baptism into death, that just as Christ was raised from the dead by the glory of the father, even so we should also walk in newness of life.

For if we have been united together in the likeness of His death, certainly we also shall be in the likeness of His resurrection,

Knowing this, that our old man was crucified with Him, that the body of sin might be done away with, that we should no longer be slaves of sin.

Jesus took all of our sins upon Himself and died on our behalf. When we ask Him into our life, God sees our old self with its sin nature and all of the sins previously committed as having been dealt with, in Christ, on that day. In other words, our old sin nature was in Christ that day and it died with Him when He died. In addition, just as Jesus rose from the dead, our new nature, that is, the born again spirit empowered by the Holy Spirit, also rises at salvation, and we are from this point to progressively live according to this nature and not the old one.

The way that we choose to live in the new nature is through faith. We discipline ourselves to no longer focus on and feed the desires that the old nature had, but to see and feed the truth of that new nature.

Romans 6:11, 12

Likewise you also, reckon yourselves to be dead to sin, but alive to God in Christ Jesus our Lord.

Therefore do not let sin reign in your mortal body, that you should obey it in its lusts.

We need to <u>see ourselves</u> as being dead to sin and that old sin nature no longer having power over our decisions, and <u>see ourselves being alive to God</u>, our spirit connected with and empowered by Him, to make right decisions in life.

Galatians 5:16-18

I say then; walk in the Spirit and you shall not fulfil the lust of the flesh. For the flesh lusts against the Spirit, and the Spirit against the flesh; and these are contrary to one another, so that you do not do the things you wish. But if you are led by the Spirit, you are not under the law.

We need to focus on and see the things of the Spirit. We are to see the truth of our new nature as revealed in the Bible. As we give attention to the things of the Spirit, Paul the apostle says in this scripture that we will not fulfill the desires of the flesh.

Romans 8:3 The Message Bible
And now what the law code asked for but we couldn't deliver is accomplished as we, instead of redoubling our efforts, simply embrace what the Spirit is doing in us.[8]

Paul is saying that we can now obey God's Word, and not sin, in a way that they could not in the Old Testament. Don't just try hard to change yourself or overcome sin in your own strength but instead, allow God's Spirit to change you from the inside out, as you keep yourself filled with the Spirit of God and the Word of God.

When I was at Bible College, a lecturer gave a good example of this, if you can overlook the ugly picture. He said there are two dogs fighting in a ring (no, I am not into dog fighting), a black dog and a white dog. Which one wins? The answer is the one that you feed the most. Feed the white dog, he said, and starve the black one and you have a rigged fight. The white dog is your spirit and the black dog is your flesh or the desires of your physical senses.

We keep a strong spirit by feeding it. As we attend to and meditate on the Word of God, stay filled with the Spirit, pray, worship, keep attending church and have great fellowship with other believers, our spirit is fed. It's like a see-saw; when your spirit is strong, your flesh or the desire to sin is suppressed. If you don't keep a strong spirit, your flesh will rise up and continue to dominate your life.

Paul also says, in Romans 8:5, that if you live according to the flesh, then it's because your mind is set there. If we want to live according to the nature of the Spirit, then we will need to set our mind on the things of God.

Romans 8:5
For those who live according to the flesh <u>set their minds</u> on the things of the flesh, but those who live according to the Spirit, the

things of the Spirit.

Romans 12:2

And do not be conformed to this world, but be transformed by the renewing of your mind, that you may prove what is that good and acceptable and perfect will of God.

The word 'transformed' is the Greek word 'metamorphoo', from which we get the word 'metamorphisis', meaning to be changed into a completely new and different species. It's the transformation of the caterpillar to the butterfly.

The day of our salvation we still outwardly look like the caterpillar. We have received God's Spirit and the potential to change, but we don't outwardly manifest the perfect being, that we've been made on the inside, in an instant. In 2 Corinthians 5:17, it says that we are new creations in Christ (or a new species). That new creation is created anew in the image of God. It looks like Jesus, thinks like Him and acts like Him. This is God's truth and, by renewing our minds on the word of God, meditating on it, we are transformed to reveal the characteristics of that new species. The more we renew our minds, the more we experience what God has for us.

So, in conclusion, we have been given a new nature and the empowerment to overcome sin and live according to the new nature. As we continue to do this and fill ourselves with the Word of God, we remove many of the hindrances to receiving healing and position ourselves on God's path to receive His promise of healing.

PICTURE

SEE YOURSELF AS DEAD TO SIN AND THAT OLD NATURE HAVING NO POWER OVER YOU. SEE YOURSELF ALIVE TO GOD, CONNECTED TO AND EMPOWERED BY HIM AND YOU WILL START TO LIVE THAT WAY.

CONCLUSION

Ephesians 2:8
For by grace you have been saved (delivered, protected, healed, preserved, made well, made whole) through faith.

God's perspective is that you have already been healed, made well and made whole, as much as you have been forgiven. Dare to believe God over the contrary symptoms, diagnoses and circumstances. Resist the thoughts of doubt and refuse to be deceived by seeing a different image to what God sees. Walk in the light as He is in the light and stay on the path of His will.

I encourage you to believe God. Meditate on His promises and see what He sees over your life. Speak the Word of His power over yourself and over those whom you are praying for.

Joshua 1:8 Amplified version
This Book of the Law shall not depart out of your mouth, but you shall <u>meditate on it</u> *day and night, that you may* <u>observe</u> (see it) <u>and do</u> *according to all that is written in it. For* <u>then</u> *you shall make your way prosperous, and then you shall deal wisely and have good success* (addition in parentheses, mine).[3]

Mark 11:23
For assuredly, I say to you, whoever says to this mountain, "Be removed and be cast into the sea", and <u>does not doubt in his</u>

heart, but believes that those things he says will be done, he will have whatever he says.

The Word conceived in your heart, to where you see what the Lord is saying to you, coupled with the Word of God in your mouth attracts 'the exceeding greatness of His power' that is to those who believe. The greatest power in the universe, that has already overcome sickness, is made available to you who believe.

1 Thessalonians 2:13
For this reason we also thank God without ceasing, because when you received the word of God which you heard from us, you welcomed it not as the word of men, but as it is in truth, the word of God, which also effectively works in you who believe.

REFERENCES

....

1. New Spirit Filled Life Bible, New King James version, Jack Hayford, executive editor. Published by Thomas Nelson Inc, Nashville, USA,2002. Used for all scriptural references unless specified otherwise.

2. Strong's Concordance/ Greek and Hebrew dictionary, James Strong. WORDsearch Corp. pp 9, 42, 125, 137.

3. The Amplified Bible, Zondervan Publishing House, Grand Rapids, Michigan, 1987. pp10, 27, 29, 32, 38, 39, 43, 80, 84, 97, 100, 103, 109/110, 130, 174, 179.

4. Complete Jewish Bible. Copyright 1998 by David H. Stern. Published by Jewish New Testament Publications, Inc. p27.

5. Young's Analytical Concordance to the Holy Bible, by Robert Young, LL.D. Eighth edition. Published by Luterworth Press, Guildford and London, 1975. p29.

6. Young's Literal Translation of the Bible, sourced from Biblegateway.com. pp 29, 32.

7. New International Version of the Bible, International Bible society, Colorado Springs, USA, 1973. pp 40, 50, 70, 72, 91, 134, 159.

8. Message Bible, Eugene H. Peterson. Navpress, Colorado Springs, Colorado, 1993. pp 43, 130, 176.

9. Vine's Complete Expository Dictionary of Old and New Testament Words. Thomas Nelson Inc, publishers, Nashville, Tennesee,1985. pp60, 89.

10. New American Standard Version of the Bible, sourced from Biblegateway.com. p116.

11. New Living Translation Bible, 2nd edition, Tyndale House Publishers, Inc, Carol Stream, Illinois, 1996. p134.

12. The Concise Macquarie Dictionary, revised edition. Published by Doubleday, Australia, Pty, Ltd. Lane Cove, Australia, 1983. p163.

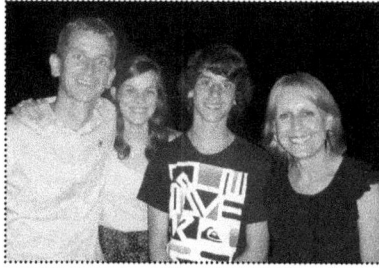

ABOUT THE AUTHOR

....

Kate Forsyth, along with her husband Richard, is a pastor at C3 Church, Oxford Falls in Sydney, Australia. They have two miracle children, Annalise and Michael.

Together Kate and Richard teach a foundational Christian teaching course and also teach in the C3 Bible College.

Over the years Kate has taught on the New Testament, the book of Revelation and 'end-times' and since 1995 on Healing. Kate and Richard run the Healing service at C3 Church, Oxford Falls where they see many people receive healing and miracles.

Her passion is to takes the truths of the Bible and make them practical and applicable to everyday life; how to have a close walk with God and experience all that He has provided for you.

Kate is available for speaking engagements.

www.ingramcontent.com/pod-product-compliance
Lightning Source LLC
Chambersburg PA
CBHW060846280326
41934CB00007B/932